THE TRIATHLETE'S TRAINING GUIDE

PLAN YOUR SEASON FROM BASE TRAINING TO RACING

THIRD EDITION

Adam Hodges

The purpose of this book is educational. It is intended to help currently healthy, physically active individuals train for their athletic goals. It is not intended to replace the advice of medical professionals. Consult with your physician to obtain medical clearance prior to beginning any exercise program. It is recommended that even experienced athletes undergo regular medical checkups and obtain medical guidance before implementing changes to an exercise program.

Alp Multisport Publications

Born in the Rocky Mountains of Colorado

alpmultisport.com

Additional titles from Alp Multisport Publications:

Run Smart: Training Tips for Runners
Adam Hodges

Copyright © 2014, 2015, 2017 Adam Hodges

All rights reserved.

Third Edition

ISBN-10: 0-9986944-0-1

ISBN-13: 978-0-9986944-0-5

DEDICATION

For those who seek to find out how far they can go

*"Only those who will risk going too far
can possibly find out how far one can go."*

~T.S. Eliot

CONTENTS

	Preface	i
PART I: FOUNDATIONAL CONCEPTS		1
1	Introduction	2
2	Exercise Science 101	9
PART II: TRIATHLON TRAINING		23
3	Your Training Intensity	24
4	Your Training Plan	39
5	Your Weekly Workouts	48
PART III: SUPPLEMENTAL TRAINING		77
6	Functional Strength	78
7	Recovery and Nutrition	103
PART IV: TRAINING PLANS & WORKOUT LIBRARY		115
8	Training Plans	116
9	Swim Workouts	162
10	Bike Workouts	193
11	Run Workouts	209
	Glossary	238
	About the Author	249

PREFACE

When preparing for a triathlon there are a lot of questions. What kind of training stress should you apply? How do you balance training with recovery? What workouts should you do and when?

What you need is a method to take the guesswork out of training. *The Triathlete's Training Guide* provides you with a simple step-by-step method to help you prepare for your triathlon goals.

Learn how to create a training plan, measure and monitor your training intensity, and schedule your weekly training. Consult chapters dedicated to functional strength training, recovery and nutrition, and key concepts from exercise science. And make use of the detailed workout library and training plans to get started.

As you begin, keep it simple. As you progress, keep in mind the basic progression of establishing and developing your base, building upon your base, and peaking for your target event. Most importantly, keep in mind that your athletic endeavors are but one piece of a larger whole that comprises your life.

The world of endurance sports is filled with many rewards. As you prepare for your events, take time to reflect on the process that gets you there—not merely the systematic training principles provided in this guide, but rather the quest of striving for a goal that challenges you physically and mentally.

For me as an athlete, the multisport lifestyle is about having fun outdoors, facing challenges, and learning more about myself in the process. I believe the challenges we engage in as athletes give us a glimpse of human potential, both on and off the race course. In this way, endurance sports act as a vehicle for discovery, personal development, and adventure. Multisport is a lifestyle. It's not about a single race or particular accomplishment; it's about the process that leads us there.

Train smart. Have fun. And above all, enjoy the journey.

PART I

FOUNDATIONAL CONCEPTS

1
INTRODUCTION

Training with a Purpose

The premise of this guide is simple: to excel in your athletic goals you need to *train with a purpose*. Training with a purpose implies a goal driven process. As an athlete training for an event, you have in mind some future destination that you wish to arrive at—a target race, a performance objective or other type of challenge. To navigate toward that destination, you need a roadmap. The roadmap is your training plan, which plots out the sections of the road you will travel with milestones along the way.

This means if you are a triathlete training for a future challenge, it is important to consider how each workout contributes to the goal driven process of preparing for your event. If you don't know why you're doing a particular workout or what training effect you're targeting, you may or may not hit the target. As a result, you may or may not be very effective at navigating toward your destination.

Fortunately, you are not the first one to train for a triathlon. Since the birth of the sport in the 1970s and with the collective knowledge surrounding human performance that has accrued in the intervening years, there is no dearth of information to guide you toward your destination. But the key to harnessing this information is to put it together into a coherent training program—that is, to take a systematic approach to training.

By acting according to a fixed plan or system, a systematic approach provides a rhyme and reason to all the miles of sweat and toil you will undertake. A systematic approach applies a consistent method that allows you to prepare for your event with greater precision. It takes you from point A to point B as effectively as possible to optimize your performance gains and increase the likelihood of success.

A systematic approach need not be a complicated approach (although it can be). It simply needs to involve a plan that starts with the end goal in mind, and schedules individual training sessions that contribute to that overarching plan. This guidebook provides you with a method to do just that. It condenses much of what I have learned over the past several decades in my training, racing, coaching, and both formal and informal studies. I attempt to present this information in an accessible manner for triathletes looking to train effectively for that next multisport challenge.

What I don't do in this guide is divulge any "newly discovered" or "hidden" training secrets. Although the information may (or may not) be new to you, it doesn't say anything that hasn't already been widely recognized by coaches, exercise physiologists and fitness professionals. There really are no hidden secrets when it comes to the basic foundations of effective training. At the end of the day, you must apply those basics and put in the work.

The principles and methods discussed in this guide pertain to any triathlete looking to prepare for an event or improve performance. Although the specific plan you create for yourself will depend upon your own unique situation, the underlying training principles remain the same for novice or veteran, short course or long course.

The ABCs of Systematic Training

The basic components of the training method found in this guide can be summarized with the following ABC mnemonic:

A: Aerobic before anaerobic
B: Build endurance along with neuromuscular speed
C: Consistent supplemental work (drills, strength, preventive care)

Aerobic before anaerobic refers to the need to establish a strong aerobic foundation before moving into the higher intensity anaerobic training zones that utilize the lactic acid system. Just as building a house requires starting with a solid foundation, so does building your fitness. Higher intensity activity is like the upper floors on a building that require a solid foundation to withstand their stress load. The more solid the foundation, the higher the building can rise. Likewise, the more solid your aerobic foundation, the faster you will eventually be able to go.

Even if you are training for short distance events that utilize a greater percentage of anaerobic energy pathways, it is important to remember that you still predominately rely upon your aerobic system as an endurance athlete. In this way, anaerobic endurance is superimposed upon one's aerobic capacity. To use another analogy, the speed you generate from tapping into the anaerobic lactic acid system is like the layer of icing on top of a cake where the cake represents your aerobic capacity. Frosting without the layers beneath it does not make for a solid cake. In the same way, focusing strictly on anaerobic training without attention to establishing a solid aerobic foundation does not make an effective endurance athlete. You may make quick gains in the short term, but at the expense of long term development. It is better to build your fitness from the ground up, establishing a strong aerobic base before moving into serious anaerobic work. This, however, does not mean you neglect speed in the true sense of term, as the next point emphasizes.

The second component—*build endurance along with neuromuscular speed*—refers to the need to develop the ability to move quickly and efficiently as you build your aerobic foundation. More specifically, by "neuromuscular speed," I mean the quick firing of muscle fibers and coordination of proper movement patterns required for economy of motion. Note that this is different than the conception of "speed" as it is sometimes used to refer to activities of a few minutes in duration where the lactic acid system is tapped.

Neuromuscular speed is achieved through short, alactic bursts—what might be viewed as "true" speed. Short sprints or hills less than 10 seconds in duration are called "alactics" because they are not long enough in duration to tap the lactic acid system. Although alactics do utilize anaerobic energy pathways, they do not stress the body the way the lactic acid system does and are therefore appropriate during base building periods. Alactics develop the body's supporting structures (e.g. muscles, ligaments, tendons) that need to be in place for higher intensity aerobic and anaerobic work down the road. In addition, alactics condition the fast-twitch and intermediate fast-twitch muscle fibers that even endurance athletes utilize during prolonged activity, and this work (along with form drills) plays an important role in improving one's economy of motion. If you can move more efficiently over a given distance, you have effectively accessed an important source of "free speed" to make you a faster athlete. This needs to be developed right alongside your aerobic endurance.

The third component—*consistent supplemental work*—refers to the need to dedicate time to activities that complement your normal sport specific workouts. This includes form drills, functional strength exercises, and preventive care to ensure flexibility and mobility. These supplemental activities need not take a great deal of time. After all, the bulk of your time is already dedicated to working out in your primary disciplines (swimming, cycling, and running). Yet even a little supplemental work can go a long way toward making you a better triathlete as long as you are consistent with it.

The R and R of Training

As athletes, we are intently focused on our training sessions—and for a good reason. If we want to swim fast or bike fast or run fast, we must swim, bike or run fast in our training. If we want to complete an Olympic distance triathlon or a full Ironman triathlon, we must build up to those distances through training sessions that increase the training load. To be successful at going farther and faster come race day, we must put in the work prior to race day. Hard work in training is a necessary component of improved fitness.

Yet hard work in and of itself is not enough to achieve improved fitness levels. Yes, hard work is necessary. But, hard work is not sufficient. Hard work must be accompanied by proper rest and recovery (the R and R of training). That is because the hard work you do during training sessions breaks down the body. It is only during the recovery phase after the training session when the body adapts to the training stress by rebuilding stronger than before. Training without adequate recovery means the body can have trouble gaining those sought after physiological adaptations, or training effects. In other words, adequate recovery is a crucial part of the overall training equation, as seen in figure 1-1.

It is easy to forget about recovery. After all, resting is a passive endeavor compared to training. You don't have to actively "do" resting like you do an interval workout. For many of us, rest seems antithetical to the hard-work mentality where pushing hard day-in and day-out is the overriding modus operandi. So it seems strange to conscientiously focus on rest and recovery. But hard work without proper recovery neglects a crucial element of the process.

> Appropriate Training + Adequate Recovery = Fitness Gain

Figure 1-1. The training equation

Begin with the End in Mind

As noted earlier, training with a purpose is a goal driven process. The goals you set help determine the roadmap you will use to navigate to your destination. So it is important to begin with the end in mind.

In addition, the process of goal setting provides an important element of the mental side of your training. Goals keep you motivated and focused on what you want to accomplish. Goals support your long term athletic development. It is no surprise that the most successful individuals in both athletics and life write down their goals.

So here are a few guidelines as you devise the goals that will drive your training program.

1. *Set long-term, intermediate, and short-term goals.* Think of the goal setting process like climbing a mountain. Your ultimate goal may be the summit (long-term goal); but to reach the summit, you need to break the climb into segments (intermediate goals) and divide those segments into individual steps (short-term goals).

2. *Keep records and evaluate progress.* Write down your goals and schedule dates for their evaluation. Feedback, whether through self-reflection or from another source such as a coach or training partner, is an essential component of the goal setting process. The feedback

you gain along the way will allow you to readjust your short-term and intermediate goals to stay on course for the long-term ones.

3. Set goals for both training and racing. It is equally important to include goals in your training as it is to have goals in your racing. Benchmark goals can help you monitor your progress on a regular basis, and daily or weekly training goals can help you stay focused on the training objectives of the moment.

4. Set goals that are difficult yet realistic. Goals should be challenging. After all, if you can easily do something, there's little need to make it a goal. Yet goals also need to be grounded in reality. Goals too far removed from an honest assessment of one's abilities can be discouraging in the long run. Goals should keep you motivated. They should challenge you to step up to that next level of performance. You may not always reach a particular goal, but that's part of the process. It's better to reach high and progress than to aim low and never really test your capabilities. The most motivating goals challenge you without defeating you.

5. Devise goals that are specific. Specific goals, rather than vague ones, will provide precision to your training program. Instead of saying, "I want to improve my marathon time" (vague), specify, "I want to qualify for the Boston Marathon next year" (specific).

6. Devise goals that are measurable. Devising goals that are specific goes hand in hand with devising goals that are measurable. If you want to qualify for the Boston Marathon, for example, that can be measured—namely, you can compare your race times to qualifying times. Measurable goals often involve time targets, e.g. "I want to run a sub-3:00 marathon."

7. State goals in the positive. Keep your eyes on where you want to go rather than where you want to avoid. Instead of saying, "I don't want to run slower than 40 minutes in the Memorial Day 10K" (negative), state, "I want to break 40 minutes for the Memorial Day 10K" (positive).

8. Keep goals under your control. As much as possible, set goals that you have control over. This means focusing more on performance- and process-related goals than outcome-related goals. *Performance goals* have to do with achieving a certain time (e.g., breaking 10 hours in the Ironman, running a 40-minute 10K). *Process goals* have to do with how you compete (e.g., keep my cadence high during the last half of my run). *Outcome goals* have to do with placement in a race (e.g., finishing on the podium). While outcome goals provide long-term motivation and many long-term goals take this form, performance and process goals help you focus on what you need to do in the intermediate and short-term, such as in the moment of the race.

9. *Own your goals.* Devise and write down goals that are agreeable to you, that you will commit to, and that you are willing to accept as your own. After all, these are your goals and should represent what you want to achieve, not what you think others want you to accomplish.

10. *Involve a support system.* Let supporters like friends, family, and training partners know what your goals are so that they can help you stay accountable to those goals and provide encouragement along the way.

2
EXERCISE SCIENCE 101

The precise training program you will follow depends upon your unique background, experience level, age, goals, time available for training, occupational stress, family commitments, and a variety of other factors that make you who you are as an individual. Yet despite the various permutations of how training can be customized to the unique situation of individual athletes, all those permutations rest upon some basic ideas from exercise science.

This chapter provides a concise overview of some of those key ideas. My aim here is to present concepts in a concise and accessible manner rather than to provide an exhaustive explication. If you are interested in learning more, I encourage you to consult any of the textbooks out there on exercise physiology. Conversely, if you are more interested in creating your training program and less interested in the scientific principles that underlie it; then you can safely skip to chapter 3 and return to this chapter as your curiosity dictates.

Stimulus-Response-Adaptation

As anyone planning to do an endurance event knows, it requires "training." But what is training? And what does this do for you exactly? Why does training make you better able to handle the rigors of an endurance event? After all, training is not simply a type of "practice" as in practicing a skill such as piano playing. Although there is skill involved in any endurance event, you are obviously interested in much more than simply acquiring skills. Through endurance training, you are looking to improve your fitness, or your ability to go faster and farther without getting tired. You are therefore interested in enhancing your body's ability to pump blood, deliver oxygen, and contract muscles.

Hans Selye, a Hungarian biologist who worked around the middle of the twentieth century, outlined a model that underlies the training process. When you train, you introduce a stimulus, or "stress" to your body. This is followed by a "response" from the body which leads to a physiological "adaptation." Selye called this *stress-response-adaptation* process the **general adaptation syndrome (GAS)**.

In discussing the importance of recovery in the introduction, I noted that the work you do during a training session breaks down the body, followed by a recovery phase during which the body rebuilds stronger than before. This is another way of describing the general adaptation syndrome. As a result of the process, you gain fitness, or the ability to perform faster and longer than before.

Many athletes take the ideas of the GAS and reason, "If training makes me stronger and faster, more training should make me even stronger and even faster." This is true as long as you are adequately recovering in between those training sessions. You can run into trouble, however, if you are comparing your training load with other athletes and simply trying to match the volume and intensity of their training programs. Crucially, *it is not the absolute training load that matters, but the training load that your body can handle.*

Overload

Discussing the GAS leads to one of the fundamental principles taught in Exercise Physiology 101: the **overload** principle. The overload principle states that any new training gain requires an appropriate training stimulus that is greater than the amount of training stress to which the body is currently adapted. Just as the name of the principle implies, you must "overload" the system to bring about a response and adaptation. Remember that the training stimulus must still be appropriate, however. It needs to be an appropriate stress to ratchet up your fitness level incrementally, rather than a stress that completely overwhelms the system and leads to overtraining or injury.

Fitness professional use the acronym FIT as a mnemonic for the key elements that comprise a training load: frequency, intensity, and time. **Frequency** refers to the number of training sessions done per week. **Intensity** refers to the effort level put forth during a training session. Time, or what is also commonly termed **duration**, refers to how long a training session lasts.

When taken together, these three elements—frequency, duration, and intensity—comprise your overall training load. Frequency and duration combine to give you training **volume**. Training volume contrasts with training **intensity**. In this way, your **training load** is comprised of volume plus intensity (see figure 2-1), or the sum total of training stress you throw at your body in its various forms.

$$\boxed{\text{Training Load} \quad = \quad \text{Volume} \quad + \quad \text{Intensity}}$$

Figure 2-1. Training load equation

Since training **volume** refers to the total amount of training you do, to quantify training volume you need to take into account the frequency of your training (i.e. how many times per week you train) plus the duration of each of those sessions. Many competitive athletes are accustomed to thinking in mileage or yardage instead of hours trained. In that case, training volume is quantified as distance rather than duration.

Training **intensity** refers to the exertion level put forth during your training sessions. Whereas volume refers to the quantity of your training, intensity deals with the qualitative nature of your training.

In sum, the overload principle states that you need to provide an appropriate training stress to achieve a fitness gain. Not enough stress and the body will fail to achieve a fitness gain. Too much stress and the body will fail to positively adapt, resulting in overtraining or injury. In other words, you need to deliver a training stimulus appropriate to your current fitness level to move you forward toward your performance goals.

Overreaching and Overtraining

According to the overload principle, you must apply an appropriate amount of stress to overload the system without overreaching or overtraining. With **overreaching**, you begin to accumulate an amount of stress that causes a temporary decrease in performance. If you continue overreaching without adequate recovery, overtraining can result. With **overtraining**, you are overburdened by stress, leading to extreme physical and mental fatigue and long term decreases in performance. Overtraining is where you dig yourself into a hole that is difficult to get out of.

It is important to note that the amount of stress that figures into the overload principle is not limited to physical training stimuli. In addition to the physical demands you place on your body during workouts, there are varying amounts of mental demands as well as stressors from other areas of your life (work, school, relationships, etc.). Every individual responds differently to varying types of stress in their lives and training. All these stressors and individual differences need to be taken into account when assessing what type of training load is appropriate for any given athlete.

Obviously, you want to apply an adaptive overload without overtraining. Once you start overtraining, it can take several weeks or even months to climb out of that hole. Extreme cases of overtraining can be season ending. Even minor cases still require unplanned time off from training to regain vitality and baseline energy levels. It is better to schedule appropriate recovery periods into your training plan and to monitor the daily signs that indicate when you need more recovery so that you can avoid overtraining in the first place.

If you are lethargic, have heavy legs or difficulty elevating your heart rate during training at increased intensity levels; then these are signs you are overtraining. If these signs continue for more than a day; then take a few days off completely followed by a few days of short, easy workouts before returning to your regular program.

With proper attention paid to how well your body is absorbing the training you throw at it, you will be able to avoid overtraining and be much more consistent with your training. This is where experience and a smart plan can help you effectively use the overload principle to attain performance gains.

Reversibility

Just as too great of a training stimulus can be detrimental to one's progression, so can be too little of a training stimulus. This follows directly from the overload principle and represents the flip side of overtraining. If you trained for and ran a marathon a few years ago and have not run since, you should not expect any carryover from that training for a marathon you decide to run on a whim next weekend. Plainly stated, the principle of **reversibility** states that inactivity leads to performance decline. Performance gains are reversed when the athlete ceases to train at a given level.

Obviously, reversibility does not mean that you can never take a break from training. Remember the earlier discussion of the general adaptation syndrome whereby proper recovery is required after overload to produce physiological adaptations. The substantial losses of fitness associated with the principle of reversibility do not occur overnight. Substantial reversals in fitness gains take one to three weeks of inactivity to achieve. But there is no need to be completely inactive for that period of time as long as you are healthy and have time to train.

Even during times when you are simply unable to train at your normal levels because other areas of your life prevent you from getting in the training you planned (e.g. work deadlines, holiday travels, unexpected illnesses, etc.), fitness can be maintained by following a reduced training schedule. The key is to not stop exercising completely.

One rule of thumb when entering into maintenance mode is to counterbalance decreased training volume with increased intensity. Aim for a short, intense workout instead of the longer workout you had planned. Also, remember that training volume is the sum of both frequency and duration. If you don't have a big block of time for that long run you originally planned, try to schedule shorter runs on back to back days or split the target duration over morning and evening runs that day. Strategies like these will allow you to maintain fitness for up to several weeks on a reduced training schedule. Just remember, something is better than nothing. The key to navigating those times of reduced training is to remain active and avoid complete inactivity.

Specificity

Earlier, I mentioned the FIT acronym used by fitness professionals. Only I left out a fourth element. The acronym is often presented as FITT with the last letter standing for type of activity—for example, swimming, biking or running. This part of the mnemonic becomes crucial when considering another fundamental principle of exercise physiology: the principle of specificity.

The principle of **specificity** states that training adaptations are specific to the system worked. For example, the best way to improve running performance is to run. If you only swam in preparation for your upcoming marathon; then your legs would not be appropriately adapted for the task of running.

It is true that endurance training results in a certain amount of **central adaptations**—that is, general adaptations to the central respiratory and cardiovascular systems. However, these improvements will only go so far in improving your sport specific performance. You also need the **peripheral adaptations** that occur in muscle groups used for a particular activity. To return to our example of the athlete that swims in preparation for a marathon, that athlete would lack the peripheral adaptations that would occur in the legs with run-specific training.

For multisport athletes, the principle of specificity means that you must train in each of the disciplines used during your races. It also means that you need to gear the type of training you do for the particular distance you will be racing. A program designed for sprint triathlons looks different than a program designed for Ironman triathlons, for example. Finally, given that everyone is an individual and responds in their own ways to different types of training, it is important that you tailor training specifically to your individual needs and situation.

Energy Systems

To sustain movement over time, we utilize energy. In our bodies, the basic currency of energy comes in the form of a high-energy compound called **adenosine triphosphate (ATP)**. Our muscles store ATP in limited amounts which can be quickly tapped for energy. The amounts are so limited that any type of activity over a few seconds in duration requires the creation of additional ATP. One way the body can immediately manufacture additional ATP is by utilizing creatine phosphate (CP) to produce a few more seconds of energy. Like ATP, only a limited amount of CP is stored in the muscles so it's only useful for short bursts of activity. Fortunately, the body is equipped with additional (although slower) manufacturing processes to supply that needed ATP.

For more pressing energy needs, the next pathway involves a process that breaks down carbohydrate stored in the muscles (glycogen) or carried in the bloodstream (glucose). As with the immediate pathways that use stored ATP and stored CP, this process occurs without the presence of oxygen. It is termed **anaerobic glycolysis**. The prefix *an-* derives from the Greek "without" while *aero-* refers to "oxygen" and *bic-* "pertaining to life." So the term *anaerobic* means life without oxygen. Since there is no oxygen present, the metabolic reaction creates an end-product called **lactate** in addition to the ATP it produces. As this energy pathway continues to produce small amounts of ATP, lactate continues to accumulate in the cells along with positively charged hydrogen atoms that make the blood acidic. If your bloodstream begins to accumulate more lactate than it can clear; then a decline in muscular performance occurs within a few minutes. Keep in mind that it's not the presence of lactate per se that causes the performance decline, but rather the acidic environment that accompanies the lactate. As anyone who has tried sprinting for a few minutes knows, sustaining that high intensity level becomes nearly impossible as your muscles start to feel like they are burning.

To continue supplying energy, the body needs a more efficient energy pathway. If oxygen is present, then that oxygen can be mixed into the metabolic reaction to form much larger quantities of ATP. In addition, this process—**aerobic oxidation** (*aerobic* meaning "life with oxygen")—can metabolize not only carbohydrate, but also fat and protein. The drawback, however, is that it takes much longer to produce the ATP than do the anaerobic pathways. As a result, your body must slow down a bit to accommodate the energy production process.

So the major energy pathways the body uses to produce energy can be characterized as either **anaerobic** (without oxygen) or **aerobic** (in the presence of oxygen). It is important to emphasize that these are not mutually exclusive pathways. Anytime you head out the door for a run, you utilize all of the available energy pathways. But you use those pathways to differing degrees depending upon the intensity at which you're exercising. The faster you run (and hence the higher the energy demands placed on the body), the more you rely upon anaerobic pathways to supply quick energy. The slower you run, the more you are able to rely upon the more efficient aerobic pathway to supply your energy needs.

As endurance athletes, we want to go as fast as possible over long distances. The better you can tap into the aerobic energy pathway while maintaining higher intensity speeds, the more successful you will be. Remember, this is because a higher reliance on the aerobic pathway provides energy while limiting the buildup of lactic acid in the blood (which can only be tolerated for so long before performance declines).

Aerobic Capacity

Endurance training results in a higher aerobic capacity. **Aerobic capacity** is a term used synonymously with **VO_2max** (volume of maximal oxygen consumption). Technically, there should be a dot above the V to indicate that one is talking about a rate. The concept refers to the highest rate of oxygen transport and use by the body during maximal physical exertion. VO_2max can be expressed in absolute terms as liters per minute (L/min), but is typically expressed relative to body weight so that comparisons among individuals can be made. Relative VO_2max is therefore expressed as milliliters per kilogram per minute (mL/kg/min). One way to improve your VO_2max is to simply become leaner.

The higher your VO_2max, or aerobic capacity, the faster you're able to move over long distances. This is because a higher VO_2max means a higher **stroke volume**—that is, for each heartbeat your heart will pump a greater amount of oxygenated blood to your muscles. Some of the top male endurance athletes in the world have recorded VO_2max scores over 80 or even 90. For example, Greg

LeMond's VO_2max was 92.5. Steve Prefontaine's was 84.4. Mountain runners Matt Carpenter and Kilian Jornet have measured 92.0 and 89.5, respectively, and track runners Jim Ryun and Steve Scott measured 81.0 and 80.1, respectively. Some top female endurance athletes have recorded scores over 70. For example, 1984 Olympic marathon champion Joan Benoit Samuelson had a VO2max of 78.6; marathoner Rosa Mota was 67.2. By comparison, anything above 55 for 20-29 year old men, above 52 for 30-39 year old men, above 50 for 40-49 year old men, above 49 for 50-59 year old men, or above 44 for men over 60 represent scores in the top 10 percentile of the male population, according to the norms provided by the American College of Sports Medicine. Likewise, anything above 49 for 20-29 year old women, above 45 for 30-39 year old women, above 42 for 40-49 year old women, above 37 for 50-59 year old women, or above 34 for women over 60 represent scores in the top 10 percentile of the female population.

Although an individual's aerobic capacity is based to an extent on genetics, it is also highly malleable. Endurance training can substantially raise one's VO_2max. And per the reversibility principle, a lack of endurance training can lower one's VO_2max. And, as you can see from the norms mentioned above, it decreases with age. Moreover, being born with a high VO_2max does not necessarily make a champion runner, cyclist, swimmer, triathlete or other type of endurance athlete. If that were the case, we might as well just all go to the lab to get our VO_2max tested and turn in the results to race organizers. Obviously, there are many factors involved in being successful at endurance events, including mental skills, nutrition, and race tactics, just to name a few. Even when it comes to VO_2max, two athletes that vary in their aerobic capacities may still possess equivalent effective aerobic capacities when taking into account economy of motion. In other words, Athlete A may achieve a 5K run time of 17 minutes with a VO_2max of 62 and fair running economy while Athlete B may achieve that same 5K time with a VO_2max of 58 and excellent running economy.

The bottom line is that laboratory recorded numbers are only a starting point. The key is knowing how to use those numbers to effectively train because endurance training will lead to better performance through many central and peripheral physiological adaptations, including an increased VO_2max, increased stroke volume (i.e. amount of blood pumped with each heart beat), increased capillary density in skeletal muscle, improved blood lipid profile, and increased lean body mass.

Lactate Threshold

Another important concept with direct implications for endurance training is the concept of the **lactate threshold (LT)**. In physiological terms, the lactate threshold (LT) refers to the point at which the rate of appearance of lactate in the blood exceeds the rate of its disappearance. In other words, when you reach lactate threshold, your bloodstream begins to accumulate more lactate than it can clear. Remember, accompanying the lactate are positively charged hydrogen atoms that make the blood acidic and contribute to muscle fatigue.

Another way to conceptualize the lactate threshold is as the boundary line between aerobic work and anaerobic work. Workloads above the lactate threshold rely more on the anaerobic pathways to produce energy, while workloads below the lactate threshold rely more on the aerobic pathway. Endurance athletes can typically hold a pace at their lactate threshold for about an hour—that duration is closer to 5 minutes for someone new to endurance training and closer to 90 minutes for an advanced endurance athlete. Yes, holding your pace at lactate threshold takes some getting used to. But learning how to push the aerobic envelope is key to successful race performance.

An important effect of endurance training is to raise your lactate threshold. Whereas before training you could run, say, 7 minutes per mile while at LT, after training the same pace would represent an intensity level below your LT. This means that you are able to go faster at a lower level of effort. In other words, you are able to stay aerobic at that given pace whereas before you moved into anaerobic territory.

Muscle Fiber Types

Endurance sports are all about movement. And to move our bodies through space and time we use muscles. Muscles operate when a signal is sent from the central nervous system (CNS) to individual cells (also called **muscle fibers**) in your skeletal muscles. As a sufficient number of muscle fibers are recruited for the task, they then contract to produce movement toward your goal.

Skeletal muscle fibers come in different flavors. When you see the difference between the leg meat and breast meat of a chicken, you know that this is literally true—dark meat tastes different than light meat. These different color patterns are a result of the chicken legs being comprised of a higher percentage of slow-twitch muscle fibers while chicken breasts contain a higher percentage of fast-twitch muscle fibers.

Slow-twitch muscle fibers—also called **Type I**—contract more slowly, just as the name implies. They are built to bring in oxygen and maximize the production of energy through the aerobic pathway. To those ends, they contain a greater number of capillaries and proteins called myoglobin to carry oxygen into the cells, along with a greater number of mitochondria which act as cellular factories for aerobic energy production. The iron-rich pigments associated with myoglobin are responsible for the color of dark meat.

Fast-twitch muscle fibers—also called **Type IIb (or IIx)**—contract more quickly and with more force than any other fiber type. They contribute substantially to shorter bursts of speed and do so through anaerobic energy production pathways. When a chicken is startled and flaps its wings to get away from a perceived threat, it recruits those fast-twitch fibers in the chest to move quickly. In contrast, the slow-twitch muscle fibers in the chicken's legs are recruited for the long duration task of walking around the farmyard all day long.

There's also a third muscle fiber type. These are called **intermediate fast-twitch**, or **Type IIa** muscle fibers. These muscle fibers possess some of the aerobic characteristics of the slow-twitch fibers as well as some of the increased contractile capability of the fast-twitch fibers.

When you decide to move your body, the first fibers to be recruited are the slow-twitch fibers. If the force demands are great enough, then the intermediate fast-twitch fibers are recruited and finally the fast-twitch fibers are called up for duty. The more force and speed you need for a given activity, the higher up the recruitment list you go.

Crucially, another factor that leads to recruiting higher up the list is fatigue. When your slow-twitch fibers become fatigued, the intermediate and fast-twitch fibers are recruited to share some of the burden. This is why even endurance athletes need to train all the fiber types. Even fast-twitch fibers are brought in to help out in endurance events as fatigue sets in. The athlete who has trained those fibers through faster paced speed work will be in a better position than the athlete who only trained by doing long aerobic workouts at lower end speeds.

Although it's true that genetics have a great deal to do with what type of fibers predominate in your skeletal muscles, endurance training can increase the aerobic capabilities of even fast-twitch fibers. A world-class sprinter may never become a world-class marathoner, but that sprinter can nevertheless improve his or her marathon time substantially through endurance training.

Periodization

As implied by the ideas discussed up to this point, improving fitness requires a balancing act between sufficient overload and adequate recovery along with training strategies that target sport specific activities as well as the various energy systems and muscle fiber types involved in those activities. So how does one put this all together?

One answer has been around since the middle of the twentieth century in an approach to training known as periodization. First used by the Soviets and soon refined by Romanian sport scientist Tudor Bompa, **periodization** involves breaking the year up into distinct training phases that build upon one another to peak an athlete for the most important competitions at the end of the season. Periodization is therefore different from doing the same type of training week-in and week-out. It is also different than randomly switching routines every month or so just for the sake of variation. What periodization contributes to training is a systematic approach to progress the athlete through successive stages over the course of the training year. Long-term progression is the goal so that the athlete arrives at the major competitions of the year in peak form.

Following the principle of specificity, periodized programs progress from general to specific, starting with general preparation and base training phases, moving through build phases, and culminating with peak training and race phases. The closer to the key race, the more specific the training becomes to target the demands of the race. After the season ends, the athlete shifts gears back to a general active recovery or transition phase before starting again with base training for the next year.

The training year as a whole is referred to as a **macrocycle**. It usually involves one or a few target races, either stacked together at the end of the year or spread apart by at least two months. The macrocycle is then divided into smaller phases of about two to six weeks in length called **mesocycles**. Each mesocycle has a particular training focus. The mesocycles are in turn comprised of smaller blocks of training that typically align with weeks. These are referred to as **microcycles**. It is quite possible to use microcycles of, say, 10 days instead of the seven day week. Such an approach could have advantages for some athletes, but for many it is easier to schedule a microcycle around the typical calendar week.

In general, training programs can vary in how they put together the pieces to create a periodization schedule. In addition, any periodization schedule is highly individual in that it needs to take into account the athlete's goals, background, and current fitness level. Yet it is widely accepted among endurance coaches that the fundamental place to begin is by establishing a strong aerobic base. Like the construction of any building, the stronger the foundation the better it can withstand loads placed on top of it. Even for endurance athletes involved in shorter events (e.g. sprint triathlons, track events down to the mile, etc.) where higher end speed is crucial, it is important to keep in mind that anaerobic endurance is superimposed upon the aerobic base. You need both for peak performance. If you are interested in long-term progression, there really are no short cuts to developing as an endurance athlete. A strong aerobic foundation is a necessity.

Part II

Triathlon Training

3
YOUR TRAINING INTENSITY

Training Intensity

A systematic approach to training involves targeted training—that is, training that targets particular training effects. And to train with precision, one needs a way to measure and monitor training intensity during workouts. This chapter provides you with a system of training zones to use with your training program. The workouts detailed later in the book prescribe intensity based on these zones.

Remember, to improve your fitness you need to add a training load to stimulate positive adaptations. In discussing training loads, I noted there are two key elements you need to keep in mind: volume and intensity. Volume is easy to measure by simply adding up the duration (or distance) of each training session. One can then talk about weekly training hours (or distances), monthly training hours (or distances), a season's training hours (or distances), etc. But training requires more than simply logging time (or distance). You also need to take into account the intensity level of the training you do.

Training intensity refers to the exertion level put forth during training. Is your workout "easy" or "hard"? Were you able to talk while doing that run or were you gasping for air? How fast did you swim that interval? These are all factors that can help characterize the intensity at which you are working. As indicated by the previous questions, intensity can be measured in a number of ways.

One of the easiest ways to dose out your effort is through perceived exertion, which means you subjectively gauge how hard you are working. Another way is to use a watch or GPS-watch to record your time over a certain distance and monitor your pace. Yet another way is to wear a heart rate monitor and use that biofeedback to measure your intensity level.

I ask the triathletes that I coach to use a heart rate monitor for their running and cycling. It provides invaluable feedback to help dial in the prescribed intensity during workouts. This is especially important if you have trouble subjectively gauging your effort. Even as you become more in tune with your body and are comfortable training by feel or only with a watch, the heart rate data from a training session can be downloaded for later analysis. This can provide insight into your response to a particular workout or progression over time. So if you're more of a data geek or want to keep closer tabs on your training, choose a heart rate monitor. But if you're drawn to the keep-it-simple approach, training by perceived exertion ("training by feel") and/or with a watch works, too. You can choose any one of these options—or, preferably, draw from a combination of these options—with the workouts provided in this guide.

Training Intensity and Lactate Threshold

The prescription of workout intensities during endurance training has typically been based on one of two physiological parameters: VO_2max or lactate threshold (see again chapter 2 for explanations of these concepts). In particular, lactate threshold has proven to be a good indicator of performance and is used by a wide array of coaches and endurance athletes as the basis for prescribing workout intensities.

The only problem is that a direct measurement of lactate threshold requires a blood sample to analyze your blood lactate levels. Although you can find portable kits to do the measurement, the process is obviously impractical for everyday training. Moreover, it is not even necessary if one can correlate lactate levels with something else, such as heart rate, pace or perceived exertion. Although heart rate, pace and perceived exertion are not direct measurements of metabolic activity, they can provide indirect approximations that are useful enough to help target your training.

In this training guide, the establishment of your individualized training zones will be based on correlating your lactate threshold with heart rate, pace, and perceived exertion. The concept of training zones is described in greater detail below.

Training Zones

Your **training zones** are the target ranges (of heart rate, pace or perceived exertion) that will be used to prescribe workout intensities. It is important to recognize that there are different nomenclatures used to talk about training zones. Some systems use fewer zones (as few as four) and some more (up to eight). Each zone corresponds to a different intensity level.

Figure 3-1 depicts a common system that uses seven zones. The first four zones correspond to aerobic intensity levels. The last three zones fall within the anaerobic range. The lactate threshold falls right at the bottom of Zone 5a, acting as the boundary between aerobic and anaerobic intensity.

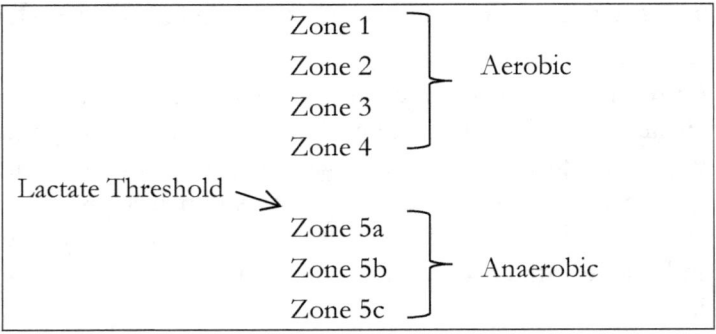

Figure 3-1. Training zones

Of the four aerobic zones, Zone 1 is used primarily for recovery and warmup or warmdown efforts. Zone 2 is the primary aerobic base building zone. This is the zone for long slow distance (LSD).

Zone 3 represents a more challenging aerobic pace. It's still well within the aerobic range but involves a peppier tempo that can be hard for the uninitiated or untrained. Think of this as aerobic tempo pace. Working in this zone is a stepping stone to tempo work that is closer to lactate threshold. But the intensity of this zone is typically too slow to gain much benefit for raising the lactate threshold and too fast to achieve the aerobic benefits of Zone 2 without causing undue wear and fatigue. Since there is little direct benefit to working in this zone, it is used sparingly and mostly avoided.

Zone 4 moves toward the lactate threshold but remains sub-threshold. This is the "comfortably hard" effort that runners refer to when talking about tempo runs.

The lactate threshold arrives at the bottom of Zone 5a, so Zone 5a corresponds to the super-threshold range. The sub- and super-threshold zones represent an important range that targets increases in the lactate threshold. Tempo workouts and cruise intervals in Zone 4 or Zones 4-5a improve lactate tolerance and decrease lactate accumulation, which enhances the ability to sustain race pace.

Zone 5b is the next step in the anaerobic range. This range corresponds to the athlete's maximal oxygen consumption, or VO_2max. Working in this zone expands aerobic capacity.

Finally, Zone 5c emphasizes anaerobic capacity. Work in this zone targets the ability to work anaerobically for events or portions of events that last a few minutes in length—such as starts, race surges, and finishing kicks.

Remember, the nomenclature used here is but one way to talk about intensity levels. It is particularly useful if you use the Training Peaks online training log to track and analyze your training. Triathlon and cycling coach Joe Friel, one of the founders of Training Peaks, uses the system; and many tools provided on Training Peaks make it easy to plug in your individual heart rate and pace data to calculate your zones according to this system.

However, other systems exist and have been adopted by different types of endurance athletes and coaches. For example, runners might be more familiar with coach Jack Daniels' system which divides training intensities into the following zones based off percentages of VO_2max: E for easy, M for marathon pace, T for threshold, I for intervals, and R for reps. Daniels uses the term "intervals" very narrowly to refer only to VO_2max or race pace intervals of 3 to 5 minutes in duration—that is, work done in what he terms the I zone. He uses the term "reps" (repetitions) to refer to work periods of less than 2 minutes at R zone pace. Daniels' E zone corresponds roughly to Zones 1-2, the M zone to Zones 2-3, the T zone to Zones 4-5a, the I zone to Zones 5a-5b, and the R zone to Zones 5b-5c.

Table 4-1. Description and uses of training zones

Description	Training Zone	Uses	Workout Characteristics
Recovery	Zone 1	Used for warmups and warmdowns, recovery workouts, and easy workouts that add to aerobic base	Easy effort
Aerobic Base (Extensive Endurance)	Zone 2	Used more than any other training zone to build the aerobic base, which allows the athlete to better metabolize fat and spare glycogen (stored carbohydrate) as a long duration energy source	Continuous effort with durations of 20 minutes up to several hours
Aerobic Tempo (Intensive Endurance)	Zone 3	Used to build intensive aerobic endurance and improve lactate tolerance	Sustained tempo for up to an hour or long intervals (e.g. 5-20 min) with a 5:1 work to recovery ratio
Sub-Lactate Threshold (LT)	Zone 4	Used to raise the lactate threshold by improving lactate tolerance and decreasing lactate accumulation, which allows the athlete to stay aerobic at faster speeds	Sustained tempo for up to an hour or long intervals (e.g. 5-20 min) with a 5:1 work to recovery ratio

(continues on next page)

Table 4-1 (cont.). Description and uses of training zones

Description	Training Zone	Uses	Workout Characteristics
Super-Lactate Threshold (LT)	Zone 5a	Used to raise the lactate threshold by improving lactate tolerance and decreasing lactate accumulation, which allows the athlete to stay aerobic at faster speeds	Sustained tempo for up to an hour or long intervals (e.g. 5-20 min) with a 5:1 work to recovery ratio
Aerobic Capacity (VO_2max)	Zone 5b	Used to increase the maximal rate of oxygen transport (aerobic capacity or VO_2max), build lactate tolerance, and increase anaerobic endurance	Work intervals of 3-7 minutes in duration with recovery interval equal to or slightly less than work interval
Anaerobic Capacity	Zone 5c	Used to improve the ability to maintain short durations of speed of up to 2 minutes in duration (starts, race surges, finishing kicks)	Work intervals up to 2 minutes in duration with recovery interval equal to or greater than work interval to allow full recovery

Regardless of the nomenclature used to talk about training zones, they all target the same energy systems on the aerobic to anaerobic continuum. It can get confusing, though, when different coaches use the same word to refer to different points on that continuum. For example, the word "cruise" as in "cruise intervals" often refers to work done at or near lactate threshold. But in Dave Scott's system, the word "cruise" characterizes what he terms the "cruise zone," which corresponds to the staple aerobic work of Zone 2 in table 4-1.

The key is to not be confused by the specific words or labels used to characterize and divide up the zones. What is most important is knowing the type of intensity level to target to gain a particular training effect. Table 4-1 summarizes the training zones used in this guide and their uses. If you know the underlying rationale of where these zones fall on the aerobic to anaerobic continuum, you can translate between the various training zone systems out there.

Training by Feel, or Perceived Exertion

One of the most basic ways to measure and monitor your exercise intensity is to subjectively gauge your effort level, or perceived exertion. To help in this task, a common tool is a **rating of perceived exertion (RPE)** scale, such as the Borg RPE scale (6-20), as seen in table 4-2, or Borg category-ratio scale (0-10). With these scales, the exerciser subjectively evaluates how they feel during a workout and points to a number on the scale to quantify their perceived exertion level.

Lactate threshold roughly corresponds to about 16, or between a hard and very hard effort on the Borg RPE scale. With this in mind, Zone 1 falls roughly between a rating of 7 and 8 on the Borg RPE scale, or an extremely light to very light effort. Zone 2 corresponds to about 9 to 11, or very light to light. Zone 3 approximates the Borg ratings of 12-14, or a somewhat hard effort. Zone 4 corresponds roughly to 15, or a hard effort. The lactate threshold arrives at the bottom of Zone 5a, which translates to about 16, or between a hard and very hard effort on the Borg RPE scale. Now in the anaerobic range, Zone 5b corresponds to 17-18 on the Borg RPE scale, or a very hard effort (bordering on extremely hard at the upper end). Finally, Zone 5c corresponds to 19-20 on the Borg RPE scale, or extremely hard to maximal exertion.

You may find the Borg RPE scale helpful, especially if you have used it before in a health club setting. But if you are looking to "train by feel," I imagine you are after something even simpler. Moreover, we need a way to translate the subjective evaluation of your effort into the training zones system discussed earlier and shown in figure 3-1. Figure 3-2 provides that key.

Table 4-2. The Borg Rating of Perceived Exertion Scale

Rating	Perceived Exertion
6	No exertion
7	Extremely light
8	
9	Very light
10	
11	Light
12	
13	Somewhat hard
14	
15	Hard
16	
17	Very hard
18	
19	Extremely hard
20	Maximal exertion

"easy"	Zone 1
"conversational"	Zone 2
	Zone 3
"comfortably hard"	Zone 4
"uncomfortably hard"	Zone 5a
	Zone 5b
"all out"	Zone 5c

Figure 3-2. Translation of perceived exertion into training zones

As you see in figure 3-2, now you simply have five perceived exertion levels to think about: easy, conversational, comfortably hard, uncomfortably hard, and all out. Think of these as cues for the type of pace you want to utilize.

An "easy" pace is the type of pace you would use during warmup, warmdown or recovery. You should certainly be able to talk to a training partner working out beside you, and could even break into song if you and your training partner are feeling musical. The "easy" designation corresponds primarily to Zone 1 (and maybe a bit into Zone 2).

A "conversational" pace means you should be able to hold a conversation while working out (but you should be working hard enough that singing would be somewhat difficult). Conversational pace corresponds primarily to Zone 2 (and into Zone 3).

With the "comfortably hard" pace, it should be difficult to hold a steady conversation. This is where those who like to talk while working out are relegated to abbreviated communicative efforts rather than a full-fledged conversation. The comfortably hard pace, also widely referred to as a "tempo" pace, corresponds to Zone 3 all the way into the bottom of Zone 5a. This is a wide range, but keep in mind that your comfortably hard pace will vary considerably depending upon where you are in your training. During your base building, your "comfortably hard" tempo work may be in Zone 3. As you progress through your training, your "comfortably hard" will move into Zone 4 and approach (and even cross over) your lactate threshold (the bottom of Zone 5a).

The "uncomfortably hard" pace moves you into the anaerobic range. To put it bluntly, anaerobic work can be downright uncomfortable. As running coach Joe Vigil has remarked, though, the key to going faster is to learn "to be comfortable being uncomfortable." In any case, the "uncomfortably hard" pace takes you into Zone 5b where you would have difficulty maintaining the pace for the same length of time as a sustained tempo session at your "comfortably hard" pace. You should be able to handle this type of pace for about 5 minutes at a time before needing a well-deserved recovery period.

Finally, the "all out" effort is simply that. It is the maximum effort that you can hold for up to a few minutes at a time. The "all out" pace corresponds to Zone 5c.

By simply focusing on these five designations, you can learn to vary your intensity to target different training effects. The workouts provided in this book prescribe intensities in terms of Zones 1-5c. If you choose to solely "train by feel" or perceived exertion instead of using heart rate and/or pace, simply aim for the designations summarized in figure 3-2. But it can be helpful to triangulate your perceived exertion with heart rate and/or pace at least until you learn to accurately "feel" what these different intensity levels are like.

Training with Pace

Pace is another means of measuring and monitoring your training intensity. The advantage of pace is that it can be easily gauged with a watch (along with distance markers) or a GPS-watch (that gives you pace). Pace works best when the terrain is relatively constant, such as on the track or in the pool. But pace can be less reliable when throwing in confounding variables, such as hills or wind. For this reason, pace tends to work best for swimming and running. Most swimming pools conveniently display a pace clock, for example. And even if you don't swim at a facility with a pace clock, you can use your watch to monitor pace. Running also works well with pace. For cycling, other methods (namely, heart rate or power) are generally preferable; so the protocols in this section only focus on how to establish your pace zones for swimming and running (although you can apply the same principle to cycling if you choose).

Your pace zones are based off your pace at lactate threshold, also known as your **threshold pace**—variously termed T-pace (for "threshold pace") or FTPa (for "functional threshold pace"). Recall from chapter 2 that you can generally maintain a pace at your lactate threshold for about an hour. But that duration may be as little as 5 minutes for untrained individuals and as close to 90 minutes for elite endurance athletes.

To establish your pace zones you need to first find out your threshold pace and then calculate your zones based on that number. This means you need to do a race or time trial where you record your time over a certain distance. The calculations involve a few different steps if you do it by hand; but you can simplify the task by using the automatic calculators found in the Training Peaks online training log or the Alp Fitness website (alpfitness.com).

For swimming, a 1,000-yd or 1,000-m time trial works well. For running, you can use the results from a 5K or 10K race or time trial. Keep in mind that the pace zones you establish work best on the same type of course on which the test was conducted. If you do your swim in a short course pool; then your swimming pace zones will help you accurately gauge your effort during subsequent workouts in a short course pool (but will be less accurate in a long course pool). Likewise, if you run a 5K time trial on a track, your running pace zones will be accurate for mainly flat terrain (but will be less helpful on a course with rolling hills). You therefore may opt to create a few different sets of pace zones for the different types of terrain or courses on which you will be regularly training.

Establishing Your Swimming Pace Zones

To determine your swimming pace zones, you first need to find your threshold pace. To do this, swim a 1,000-yd or 1,000-m time trial (TT) at a race-level effort. This means you should go into the TT well rested and ready to go as fast as you can over that distance. Record your time for the TT and then divide that time by 10 to find your pace per 100. Typically, this works out to be a good approximation of your threshold pace.

Write this number in table 4-3 where it says "T-pace." From there, calculate your pace in the other cells of the right column by adding or subtracting the number of seconds indicated. To create a range, add and subtract 2-3 seconds from the number you come up with for each cell. This will give you a good estimate of the pace you want to target when working in the different training zones.

Instead of figuring the pace zones by hand, you can also use the automatic calculator found on the Alp Fitness website (alpfitness.com) or the Training Peaks online training log.

Keep in mind that for the calculations of your swimming pace zones to be accurate, the results of the TT need to represent a race-level effort. In my experience coaching swimmers of different levels, I have found that a 500 TT often works better for novice swimmers who are unaccustomed to "racing" longer distances. In such cases, you can find your pace per 100 based on the results of a 500 TT. On the other hand, experienced swimmers will be able to hold a pace slightly faster than threshold pace for a 1,000-yd/m time trial. If that's you, you may use a longer time trial (e.g. 1.5-km or 1.2-mile) or convert your 1,000-yd/m time to an equivalent performance of a longer distance to better approximate your threshold pace. Once you have your threshold pace; then use table 3-3 to determine your target paces for the different training zones.

Table 3-3. Pace zones for swimming based on threshold pace

Swimming Pace Zone	Swimming Pace (pace per 100)
1	Very easy effort
2	T-pace + 10 sec
3	T-pace + 5 sec
4	T-pace
5a	T-pace
5b	T-pace – 5 sec
5c	Maximum effort

Establishing Your Running Pace Zones

To determine your running pace zones, you first need to find your threshold pace. To do this, you can either run a solo time trial or use the results from a recent race, such as a 5K, 10K or another distance up to a half marathon.

Remember that threshold pace is generally the pace you can hold for about an hour. This means if you use a 5K (for most runners) or even a 10K (for many runners), your "race pace" at those distances will be faster than threshold pace. You have a few different options for calculating your threshold pace to account for this difference.

First, divide your time by the distance to obtain your average pace for that distance. Next, if you ran a 5K, multiply that average pace by 1.07. If you ran a 10K, multiply the average pace over the 10K by 1.01. For most people, the result will be a good approximation of your threshold pace. Once you have that number, use the percentages in table 3-4 to calculate your running pace zones.

Another option for calculating your threshold pace is to plug your result for the 5K or 10K or other distance into a calculator to determine an "equivalent running performance" of closer to an hour.

You can find an equivalent running performances calculator on the Alp Fitness website (alpfitness.com). Take the average pace of that equivalent performance in the one hour range and use that as your threshold pace. Then use the percentages in table 3-4 to calculate your running pace zones. Yet another option is to use the automatic calculator found in the Training Peaks online training log.

Table 3-4. Pace zones for running based on threshold pace

Running Pace Zone	Running Pace (pace per mile)
1	< 129% of FTPa
2	114-129% of FTPa
3	106-113% of FTPa
4	101-105% of FTPa
5a	97-100% of FTPa
5b	90-96% of FTPa
5c	> 90% of FTPa

Beyond formulas and calculators, remember the underlying premise of what you are looking to find. Namely, your functional threshold pace represents a pace you can hold for about an hour (for most athletes). If you are new to endurance training, this duration will be shorter—in that case, simply using the results of a 5K or 10K race level effort may work. Or, if you are a sub-1:20 half marathon runner; then using the average pace from a half marathon could work.

Training with Heart Rate

Another option you have for gauging your intensity during training is a heart rate monitor. Heart rate training is particularly useful for running and cycling. The more the terrain varies the less accurate pace is as an indication of exercise intensity. For example, if you are running uphill, your intensity level will be much higher for a given pace than for that same pace run on a flat surface. Your heart rate monitor will better reflect the difference in exercise intensity between those two efforts than your watch. So heart rate can be a much more precise method for monitoring your effort during a workout.

As with the other measurement tools, to effectively use heart rate you need to correlate it with your lactate threshold. As with the pace zones, your heart rate zones are specific to the activity. So you will have different heart rate zones for each discipline in which you train.

Your lactate threshold heart rate (LTHR) for cycling is typically 5 to 10 beats lower than your LTHR for running, so you can easily estimate one from the other if you do not have sport specific tests for both running and cycling. But the most accurate way to determine your sport specific training zones is to use sport specific results.

To determine your heart rate zones, you will need to do a race or solo time trial. Any race lasting up to an hour can be used. Or you can do a time trial of 20 to 30 minutes in duration. A fairly flat course should be used so that a consistent effort can be maintained over the distance. Whether in a race or solo time trial effort, you will need to record your average heart rate. It's also good to note your perceived exertion level, as well as other conditions (such as weather, pre-race meals, recent sleep patterns, etc.) in your training log.

For a race, simply note your average heart rate over the distance. For a 30 minute solo time trial, take your average heart rate for the last 20 minutes. For those new to endurance training, these numbers are generally a good estimation of your LTHR. For more experienced athletes, your effort over these shorter distances will be slightly higher than your LTHR (which, remember, corresponds to a race pace effort of about an hour in duration). In that case, divide the average heart rate from a race by 1.04 and the average heart rate from a short solo time trial by 1.02. The number you come up with is your LTHR. Use the percentages in table 3-5 to calculate your heart rate zones. As with the pace zones, you can also use the automatic calculators found on the Alp Fitness website (alpfitness.com) or in the Training Peaks online training log.

Once you know your sport specific training zones, you are ready to put them to use in your training program. The next two chapters examine how to develop that program, starting with a big-picture look at your season and then how to implement your training through the different phases of the season.

Table 3-5. Heart rate zones for running and cycling based on percentage of lactate threshold heart rate (LTHR)

Heart Rate Training Zone	Running (percentage of LTHR)	Cycling (percentage of LTHR)
1	66-84%	66-80%
2	85-90%	81-89%
3	91-95%	90-93%
4	96-99%	94-99%
5a	100-102%	100-102%
5b	103-106%	103-106%
5c	106-111%	106-111%

4
YOUR TRAINING PLAN

As discussed at the end of chapter 2, a *periodized* training plan divides the year into distinct training phases. The training phases are like stepping stones that build upon one another to peak you for your target race or races. There are three basic steps to building your fitness from the ground up. First, you establish and develop your base. Second, you build upon your base. Third, you peak for your target race. Establishing and developing a solid base, and then building upon that base leads the way to peak performance. This chapter discusses how to prioritize your races and create your training plan with the base-build-peak progression in mind.

Prioritizing Your Races

Before you put together your training program, you must look at the big picture and determine your destination before mapping out the training phases and scheduling weekly workouts. In other words, you want to begin with the end in mind by pinpointing your top competitive priorities and working backwards on the calendar to create your training plan.

To determine your most important race or races of the year, write down your race schedule for the upcoming season and prioritize those races as follows.

A-priority races: These are the one to three most important races of the season. Training will be designed around these races to allow you to peak for them. Ideally, these will occur together in a two or three week time period; or, they may be separated by a few months or more.

B-priority races: These can be up to six races of lesser importance. These are races you want to do well at, but will not peak for. Training will be designed to give you a few days of rest prior to them, but not a complete taper as with the A-races you will peak for.

C-priority races: These are races done as tests, hard workouts, experience, fun, etc. You will "train through" these races. Deciding whether or not to do one of these races may be left up to the week (or day) of the race.

Table 4-1. A sample race schedule

Date	Race	Priority
June 14	Local 10K	C
August 9	Dip N' Dash	B
August 30	State Triathlon	A

Table 4-1 illustrates a summer race schedule that features three races: a low priority 10K to be used as training on June 14, an intermediate priority swim-run event on August 9, and the top priority triathlon on August 30.

Here, the athlete wants to peak for the State Triathlon at the end of the summer, and therefore works backwards from this race to plot out a 15-week training plan as illustrated in table 4-2. The Local 10K falls at the end of week 4 and the Dip N' Dash takes place at the end of week 12. The plan culminates with the peak event at the end of week 15.

Overview of the Training Phases

As noted earlier, you will periodize, or "chunk" your training into three basic phases: the base phase, the build phase, and the peak phase. These three phases represent the base-build-peak progression that takes you to your target race.

During the base phase, the bulk of your training consists of lower intensity aerobic work as you increase your training volume. This establishes your aerobic foundation or "base" and enhances the body's ability to metabolize fat as an energy source. As you build your endurance during base training, you also want to develop your neuromuscular speed through short bursts of speed of less than 10 seconds in duration with ample recovery between. These "alactics" can easily be incorporated into your endurance workouts, along with drills to emphasize efficiency of movement. The purpose of the base phase is to increase your aerobic capacity and prepare your body for the rigors of higher intensity training and racing down the road.

Table 4-2. A sample racing season with races mapped out

Week	Race	Priority
1		
2		
3		
4	Local 10K	C
5		
6		
7		
8		
9		
10		
11		
12	Dip N' Dash	B
13		
14		
15	State Triathlon	A

Whereas the base training phase is marked by increases in training volume, the build phase is marked by increases in training intensity while volume levels off or decreases. During the build phase, more time is spent on lactate threshold work. In addition, anaerobic work of varying intensities is added—especially for advanced athletes or those targeting shorter events.

As the target race approaches, you move into the peak phase of training. The peak phase can be thought of as a more specialized build period where higher intensity (rather than volume) is emphasized. As the race approaches, volume decreases while intensity is maintained or raised. This stepping down in volume helps you rest and taper while the intensity sharpens you for the target race.

If you have more than one top priority race scheduled at the end of the season, a few weeks of peak training might then be followed by two to three weeks in race mode where peak form is maintained between weekly races with high intensity/low volume workouts.

After the season ends, you transition into an active recovery phase. Although time off from the sport is certainly advisable, it's better to avoid more than a week or two of complete inactivity. Aim for light, easy workouts to remain physically active. To take a mental break from your competitive sports, engage in other activities you enjoy such as hiking, surfing, skiing, basketball, tennis, etc. The point is to refresh your mind and body while maintaining general fitness. After all, aren't you doing this because you enjoy living a healthy, active lifestyle? Use your out-of-season training time to explore that lifestyle further. The off-season is also a good time for multisport athletes to focus on a single sport for a change of pace—either to develop a weak link in triathlon or to learn more about one's potential in a single discipline through focused training and racing in that sport.

As the off-season moves toward a new season's base phase, some general preparation work should be done to ensure you hit the ground running when base training starts. A prep phase allows you to transition from an active recovery period after the end of your previous season and prepares the body to return to regular training. Think of the prep phase as a lower volume pre-base training period. Most people who enjoy living a multisport lifestyle easily maintain a baseline level of activity in between seasons, and this acts as a type of prep phase prior to a new season's base training. The key point is that you need to be ready to handle the training volume scheduled for your first week of the new season's base phase so you're not starting from zero.

Choosing Your Periodization Schedule

As you divide your training year into phases, you also need to consider how to chunk your training within those phases. Here, it is necessary to revisit the terminology associated with periodization introduced at the end of chapter 2.

Recall that a macrocycle encompasses your training year as a whole. For the purpose of illustration, let's consider the 15 week training plan in table 4-2 as this athlete's macrocycle. The next step is to divide those 15 weeks (the macrocycle) into intermediate training periods (or mesocycles). From one perspective, these mesocycles could simply refer to the general phases discussed earlier (base, build, and peak).

However, it is helpful to chunk training into distinct blocks that provide a few weeks of increasing volume and/or intensity followed by a recovery week. For example, a four week block of training, or mesocycle, may involve three weeks (each week is a microcycle) of increasing volume and/or intensity followed by one week dedicated to recovery. This is known as a 3-up/1-down periodization pattern. The recovery week builds extra time into the schedule to allow the athlete to absorb the previous training. Keep in mind this is not a week off from training, but merely a week (or partial week) with reduced volume and intensity to give the body a chance to rebuild stronger than before (recall that fitness gains occur during recovery not actual training!). The built-in recovery time ensures that positive adaptations (rather than negative adaptations that lead to injury) are achieved with the training.

Another option for a periodization schedule is a 2-up/1-down pattern, which involves two weeks of increasing volume and/or intensity followed by one week with extra recovery built in. The 2-up/1-down pattern works well for athletes new to training, athletes prone to injury, and older athletes.

Do you need to schedule an entire recovery week at the end of each of these mesocycles? Maybe not. Advanced athletes and younger athletes are often able to get away with simply scheduling a few extra recovery days. But athletes new to training and those prone to injury and overtraining generally benefit from scheduling a full recovery week.

Assess your own background and situation to decide how to periodize your training. The possibilities are certainly not limited to the 3-up/1-down or 2-up/1-down schedules discussed here. But if you cannot match the quality of the training prescribed in a new mesocycle; then you may not be adequately recovered from the previous mesocycle. This is a clear sign that you need to pay more attention to recovery and reduce volume/intensity during scheduled down weeks. The periodization pattern you ultimately choose should be based on your background, current fitness level, goals, and response to training.

Table 4-3. A sample training plan divided into training blocks

Week (microcycle)	Block (mesocycle)	Race	Priority
1	Base 1		
2			
3			
4	(recovery)	Local 10K	C
5	Base 2		
6			
7			
8	(recovery)		
9	Build		
10			
11			
12	(recovery)	Dip N' Dash	B
13	Peak		
14			
15		State Triathlon	A

In the example of the 15 week training plan seen earlier, let's use a 3-up/1-down pattern. This chunks the training into two base training blocks, one build block, and a final peak block of three weeks, as seen in table 4-3. Note that the lesser priority races fall at the end of recovery weeks. This strategy allows the athlete to recover a bit from previous training and use the races to test fitness gains. Likewise, if the athlete didn't have races scheduled at the end of these down weeks, benchmark tests could alternatively be scheduled into the training plan.

Filling in the Details of the Overall Plan

With the base-build-peak progression sketched out into training blocks, next assign your weekly training hours. Setting these numbers in advance allows you to manipulate training volume systematically. This helps to avoid doing too much one week and not enough on other weeks. It doses out your training in a manner that allows you to consistently ratchet up your fitness.

Crucially, setting the number of weekly training hours is dependent upon your background and current fitness level. You must start from where you currently are, and progress from there. Simply choosing training hours based on what someone else does or what you think you need to do for a given race distance overlooks your own unique situation.

Consider the average weekly training hours you put in over the previous season. That is your starting point. If you are looking to increase your training hours this season, use the 10 percent rule of thumb and increase your training hours accordingly. Although merely a "rule of thumb," avoiding big jumps in training volume by limiting increases to about 10 percent from year to year is a safe way to proceed. It is best to take a long term view toward your progression in the sport and increase volume gradually over several years.

Trying to match what top athletes are doing can often lead to burn-out or injury. It takes elite athletes many years to work up to the training load they use. Likewise, trying to jump into the training volume required to race a long course event during your first season in the sport is not advised. Look long term and plan your progression over a few years rather than trying to do it all in one season. Start where you are currently.

With this in mind, input an appropriate number of training hours in the first week of your initial base training block—that is, an amount appropriate to your current fitness level. This means your pre-base training should sufficiently prepare you to step into this amount of training. From there, increase your hours by about 10 percent per week on the "up" weeks of each training block. For the "down" weeks, lower the volume by about a third to a half. In the build periods, your training hours level off or decrease as intensity builds. An example of this progression of weekly training hours can be seen in table 4-4.

Table 4-4. A sample training plan

Week	Block	Hours	Race	Priority
1	Base 1	8		
2		9		
3		10		
4		6	Local 10K	C
5	Base 2	10		
6		12		
7		14		
8		8		
9	Build	9		
10		9		
11		9		
12		6	Dip N' Dash	B
13	Peak	8		
14		6		
15	Race	5	State Triathlon	A

With the weekly total training hours outlined, you can then specify weekly targets for swimming, cycling, and running. You can also schedule in training hours for supplemental work, such as strength and flexibility training. A rule of thumb for balancing your training across the three disciplines is to dedicate about 20 percent of your training time to swimming, 50 percent to cycling, and 30 percent to running. Keep in mind this is a general rule and works well for athletes who are fairly well balanced across the disciplines. But everyone has their own strengths and weaknesses, so adjust these ratios depending upon your own needs. A mantra triathletes often use is *train your weaknesses and race your strengths*. If you are a weak cyclist but a strong runner, you may need to dedicate more training time to cycling. The point is to focus your training where you will reap the most rewards come race day, rather than simply indulging in what you are best at or what you like to do the most.

The point about "where you will reap the most rewards come race day" also needs to take into account how race splits in each discipline will contribute to your overall performance. You might be able to take a minute off your 1.5K swim time if you spend 5 hours extra in the pool each week. But if that takes away from, say, the time you are able to spend cycling, which translates into a slower bike split by 4 minutes; then your overall triathlon performance is worse off. It is not uncommon, for example, for some Ironman triathletes with a good swimming background to swim little more than many do to prepare for a sprint distance triathlon. They may lose a few minutes over what they could potentially swim for 2.4 miles, but in turn may gain tens of minutes or more by focusing their training on the bike and run. The key point is to know where your own strengths and weaknesses lie and where you should focus your training to gain the most benefit come race day.

Now that you have a big picture overview of your training season, the next chapter discusses how to implement your training.

5
YOUR WEEKLY WORKOUTS

With your individualized training zones established (chapter 3) and the outlines of your training plan on the calendar (chapter 4), now it is time to implement the plan by scheduling your weekly workouts. This chapter examines the types of workouts to schedule throughout the base-build-peak progression.

Creating Weekly Schedules

Recall that your training plan consists of intermediate level training blocks (mesocycles). Each week within those training blocks represents a smaller chunk of training (microcycle). These are commonly referred to as training "weeks" because they typically correspond to a 7-day calendar week. However, keep in mind that you could just as easily use microcycles of 10 days instead (or any number of days you choose). Most people adopt the typical 7-day training week because that is how we schedule the rest of our lives; so it is therefore easier to schedule our training that way, too.

As you schedule workouts over the week (microcycle), aim to balance workloads and recovery as you juggle training with other life activities and commitments. This means balancing harder days with easier days to ensure you are recovering adequately in between the key workouts. Just as you schedule extra recovery days at the end of each mesocycle, you want to take a similar approach to your weekly training schedule. If you do not like to take a full day off each week; then at least try to schedule an active recovery day to provide a physical and mental break.

Another consideration for triathletes is the need to space the different disciplines throughout the week with an eye toward avoiding too many consecutive days off from any one sport. A good rule of thumb is to avoid more than three consecutive days without training any one of the disciplines. If you do two swims, two bikes, and two runs each week, this is easy to accomplish. A schedule of three workouts per discipline per week with no more than two days off from any one discipline provides even more consistency.

Remember that to achieve a certain training volume over the course of the week, you have two variables to manipulate: *frequency* of sessions and *duration* of sessions. For example, two sessions of 1.5 hours each will give you the same training volume as three 1-hour sessions. Consider spreading out your weekly training volume over multiple sessions rather than trying to stack that volume into fewer sessions. One advantage of this approach is that your body better handles greater volume when it is spread out over multiple sessions, leaving you less prone to injury and overtraining. Another advantage is that you are better able to maintain form by limiting the number of consecutive days off from any single discipline. And if you are working to improve your skills in a discipline, you will benefit from an increased frequency of sessions—for example, getting in the water more frequently will benefit you if you are new to swimming.

Another useful strategy for triathletes is to schedule the long swim, long bike, and long run on back to back days and in that order. This mimics the sequence in which the disciplines are encountered in a race, providing an important element of race specific training where you learn to deal with fatigue that is carried over from one sport to another—especially from the bike to run on back to back days.

Establishing and Developing Your Base

During base training, your dual focus is to build endurance and foster neuromuscular speed. This means your training will primarily consist of endurance sessions in Zone 2, or "conversational pace." Often termed "long slow distance" (LSD), this work is foundational to developing your aerobic system. Yet this work needs be complemented with training to develop neuromuscular speed. This simply involves incorporating several short bursts of speed of less than 10 seconds in duration into one or more endurance workouts each week. The short sprints are punctuated by ample recovery in between. These "alactics" stimulate the firing of fast-twitch muscle fibers without tapping into the lactic acid system. Note that this is "pure speed," as opposed to the notion of speed as it is sometimes used to refer to activities of a few minutes in duration that do tap into the lactic acid system. In addition, you should supplement your swim, bike and run training with functional strength work (see chapter 6) and form drills (see the workout library at the end of the book) to further foster proper neuromuscular patterning for economy of movement. As your base training progresses, you can add in work closer to your lactate threshold—that is, tempo work and cruise intervals in Zones 3-4, or "comfortably hard" pace. With this overview in mind, let's look at some of the key workouts during base training in more detail.

Endurance Workouts

Endurance workouts form the bulk of your training time. This is true across the base-build-peak progression; but endurance workouts are particularly important during base training because this is your starting point for building your fitness.

An endurance workout consists of a continuous effort in Zone 2 or at "conversational" pace for durations of 20 minutes up to several hours (depending upon the sport, the athlete, and the event being trained for). The purpose of these workouts is to build your aerobic base by developing the ability to better metabolize fat and spare glycogen (stored carbohydrate) as a long duration energy source. See figure 5-1 for a summary of this type of workout; and see the swim, bike and run workouts in chapters 9, 10 and 11 for specific examples.

One endurance workout each week is typically designated as the "long" session. The long swim, long bike or long run simply represents the longest session in each of these disciplines for the week. As base training progresses, the duration of the weekly "long" training session is gradually increased during the "up" weeks of your training. This is the case for at least the long bikes and long runs. For many triathletes—especially those training for short course events—

there is little difference in duration between the "long" swim and other swim sessions.

During your endurance runs, focus on keeping a high cadence. Elite runners average 28 to 30 left foot strikes per 20 seconds (84 to 90 per minute). Aim to improve upon your personal baseline to develop good neuromuscular patterns and running form. During the endurance bikes, focus on keeping your cadence at 90 revolutions per minute or more throughout the ride (use a cadence sensor on a bike computer or Garmin training device for feedback).

Endurance Workout

When:	All training phases, especially base training
Why:	To build the aerobic base by developing the ability to better metabolize fat and spare glycogen (stored carbohydrate) as a long duration energy source
What:	Continuous effort in Zone 2 or "conversational" pace for durations of 20 minutes up to several hours
How:	Use heart rate, pace or perceived exertion to monitor intensity

Figure 5-1. Summary of the endurance workout

Although you can certainly do your endurance swims in open water (if available) or for a prescribed amount of continuous time in a pool, you can also break up the swims into intervals. This could be anything from 100s up to 1,000s, punctuated with rest intervals of about 10 seconds for each 100 swum during the work interval. For example, you could do a set of 15 x 100 with 15-20 seconds rest. Or you could do 3 x 500 with 50 seconds rest. Or perhaps 2 x 1000 with 90 seconds rest. See the sample workouts at the end of the book for more ideas.

The long endurance session each week provides you with a designated day to focus on a single session of greater volume. As you progress through your base training, this long session will increase in duration (at least for the bikes and runs). Start at your current fitness level and gradually add duration from there. Generally speaking, you can follow the 10 percent rule of thumb to gradually increase the duration of your long session until you hit your maximum targeted volume in your training plan for that type of workout. The precise volume you target for the long session in each discipline will be determined by the type of event you are training for. In other words, your long sessions will be longer for long course events (e.g. Ironman and Ironman 70.3 triathlons) than they would be for short course events (i.e. sprint and Olympic distance triathlons). For short course training, you can top out at 2 to 2.5 hours for long bikes and 1.5 hours for long runs. There is a definite benefit, though, to being out there for that amount of time even for short course training.

Endurance Workouts with Alactics

As noted earlier, your focus during base training centers on building endurance along with neuromuscular speed. To work on developing neuromuscular speed, you can incorporate several short, alactic bursts of less than 10 seconds in duration into an endurance workout. These are called "alactics" because they are not long enough in duration to tap the lactic acid system. Although alactics do utilize anaerobic energy pathways, they do not stress the body the way the lactic acid system does and can be used throughout base training to develop the body's supporting structures (e.g. muscles, ligaments, tendons) that need to be in place for higher intensity aerobic and anaerobic work down the road. In addition, alactics condition the fast-twitch and intermediate fast-twitch muscle fibers that even endurance athletes utilize during prolonged activity; and this work (along with form drills) plays an important role in improving your neuromuscular patterning for economy of motion.

Once you are warmed up, add a handful of short accelerations to an endurance workout. Start off easy and gradually pick up your pace until you're at full speed. Hold top speed for up to 10 seconds; then wind it back down. These are "feel good" sprints—you want to feel good going fast. Focus on good form. Don't worry about time or heart rate during the accelerations. Swim, bike or run for 2 to 3 minutes between each acceleration or until you feel fully recovered and ready for the next one. See figure 5-2 for a summary of this type of workout; and see the swim, bike and run workouts at the end of the book for specific examples.

<u>Endurance Workout with Alactics</u>
When: All training phases, especially base training
Why: To build the aerobic base and neuromuscular speed
What: Continuous effort in Zone 2 or "conversational" pace for durations of 20 minutes up to several hours. Throughout the workout, add 4-16 short accelerations where you build to maximum speed and hold it for up to 10 seconds. Start off easy and gradually pick up your pace until you're at full speed. Hold it for up to 10 seconds; then wind it back down. These are "feel good" sprints—you want to feel good going fast. Focus on good form. Don't worry about time or heart rate during the accelerations. Swim, bike or run for 2-3 minutes between each acceleration or until you feel fully recovered and ready for the next one.
How: Use heart rate, pace or perceived exertion to monitor intensity

Figure 5-2. Summary of the endurance workout with alactics

<u>Recovery Workout</u>
When: All training phases
Why: To aid recovery, add to your training volume and loosen you up for the key workouts of the week
What: Workout done in Zones 1-2 or at "easy" to "conversational" pace. Usually 20-30 minutes in duration, but can be longer.
How: Use heart rate, pace or perceived exertion to monitor intensity

Figure 5-3. Summary of the recovery workout

Recovery Workouts and Drills

"Recovery" workouts are done in Zone 1, or "easy pace" to provide a physical and mental break from the harder days. These workouts are typically quite short in duration—enough to loosen up and get the blood flowing. Nevertheless, they also add to your overall training volume. The key to a successful recovery workout is to avoid the temptation to go faster than recovery pace (even if you're feeling good); otherwise you sabotage the point of the workout. See figure 5-3 for a summary of this type of workout; and see the swim, bike and run workouts at the end of the book for specific examples.

Recovery workouts—as well as other endurance workouts—provide a great opportunity to incorporate drills into your training. Athletes that regularly incorporate drills into their training are better able to recruit muscles needed for the task, leaving them less injury prone. And when the going gets tough, they are more efficient. Given that an improvement to economy of motion is just as good as an improvement in VO_2max when it comes to that final number on the stopwatch, it only makes sense to squeeze as much "free speed" out of your performance as possible. The key to developing good form is to ingrain proper movement patterns into your muscle memory so that they become automatic; and proper movements can be trained through drills. With proper movement patterns instilled as the default setting, you will be better prepared when fatigue threatens to break down your form.

Drills should be introduced into your workouts at the beginning of your base training. Throughout the rest of your training phases, you can continue to incorporate drills into your recovery or endurance workouts. Form work is particularly important for swimming and running. See the swim, bike and run workouts in chapters 9, 10 and 11 for drills specific to each discipline.

Establish Your Base: Early Base Training Sample Schedules

With these basic workouts in mind, let's look at some sample early base training schedules that draw from these workouts. Tables 5-1, 5-2, and 5-3 illustrate sample weekly schedules for the early stages of base training for athletes doing two, three, and four workouts per discipline per week, respectively.

In table 5-1, the triathlete has scheduled two workouts per discipline for the week. One of those workouts is dedicated to a longer endurance session. Incorporated into that endurance workout are alactics. The second workout is designated as a recovery workout where the triathlete also focuses on drills. One day is designated as a rest day, or a day off from training.

Table 5-1. Sample early base training week with 2 workouts/discipline

Day	Discipline	Workout
Monday	SWIM	Recovery w/drills
Tuesday	BIKE	Recovery w/drills
Wednesday	RUN	Recovery w/drills
Thursday	--	
Friday	SWIM	Endurance w/alactics
Saturday	BIKE	Endurance w/alactics
Sunday	RUN	Endurance w/alactics

In table 5-2, the triathlete has scheduled three workouts per discipline for the week. With workouts over seven days, this requires doubling up on three days while taking one day completely off from training. The long swim, long bike, and long run are scheduled on back to back days over the weekend. This mimics the order in which the events are encountered in a race. Even though these workouts are not performed on the same day (as with a race), the athlete still must deal with fatigue that is carried over from one day to the next. This particularly pertains to the long run on Sunday, which is scheduled the day after the long bike.

The second workout for each discipline during the week is a recovery workout. The remaining workout is an endurance workout that incorporates drills and alactics. On Thursday, a bike and a run are scheduled. Ideally, this will be done as a "brick" workout, which means the run is done immediately after the bike. This allows the athlete to practice running off the bike. For the uninitiated, running off the bike often results in wobbly legs. But with practice during training, the odd feeling of doing one after the other becomes more familiar and easier to handle. You can also use these workouts as an opportunity to work on your bike to run transition skills. But even if you don't set up a transition area with your equipment all laid out as in a race, aim to limit your transition time to around 10 minutes during bike-run bricks.

Note that on Tuesday in table 5-2, the swim and bike workouts are scheduled in the same order encountered during a race. Although the logistics of arranging your workouts around other life commitments often dictate how you need to arrange multiple workouts throughout a given day, it can be helpful to mimic the order in which you encounter the events during a race—even when you do not perform the workouts as a brick. Here, the swim is done early in the day and the bike ride done later in the day—likewise for the swim and run scheduled on Wednesday. When not targeting a brick workout, it is a good idea to allow several hours in between workouts. This gives you time to recover and allows you to get more out of each workout as a result.

Table 5-2. Sample early base training week with 3 workouts/discipline

Day	Discipline	Workout
Monday	--	--
Tuesday	SWIM	Endurance w/drills & alactics
	BIKE	Endurance w/drills & alactics
Wednesday	SWIM	Recovery
	RUN	Endurance w/drills & alactics
Thursday	BIKE/RUN	Recovery
Friday	SWIM	Long
Saturday	BIKE	Long
Sunday	RUN	Long

In table 5-3, the triathlete has scheduled four workouts per discipline for the week. The fourth workout involves another endurance workout.

Table 5-3. Sample early base training week with 4 workouts/discipline

Day	Discipline	Workout
Monday	SWIM	Recovery
Tuesday	SWIM	Endurance w/drills & alactics
	BIKE	Endurance w/drills & alactics
Wednesday	BIKE/RUN	Endurance
	SWIM	Endurance
Thursday	RUN	Endurance w/drills & alactics
	BIKE	Recovery
Friday	SWIM	Long
	RUN	Recovery
Saturday	BIKE	Long
Sunday	RUN	Long

In sum, during early base training, one key workout each week should be a longer endurance session. Another workout should be dedicated to recovery. Alactics and drills can be added to either of these or a third endurance session. Additional workouts added to the schedule should consist of endurance and/or recovery sessions. The aim of the training is to build that all important aerobic foundation.

Aerobic Tempo and Threshold Workouts

As you progress in your base training, you begin to add work closer to your lactate threshold. This involves work done at the "comfortably hard" pace of Zones 3-4. Recall from chapter 3 that Zones 3-4 remain in the aerobic range below your lactate threshold. Think of Zone 3 as a low-level sub-threshold zone and Zone 4 as a high-level sub-threshold zone. Remember, your lactate threshold occurs right at the bottom of Zone 5a; so Zone 5a represents a super-threshold zone.

In the workouts at the end of the book, I label Zone 3 workouts as "aerobic tempo" and Zone 4 as "threshold." But here, I refer broadly to both as threshold workouts. This is because the workout design is the same regardless of the specific zone you target (Zone 3, Zone 4 or Zones 4-5a).

Threshold work involves either a bout of sustained tempo for up to an hour or cruise intervals that break up your time at tempo using a 5 to 1 work to recovery ratio. In other words, to use running as an example, you can do a tempo run where you up your intensity to a "comfortably hard" pace for 30 minutes. Or, you can do a set of, say, 3-4 cruise intervals where you run at "comfortably hard" pace for 8 minutes followed by 2 minutes at an "easy" or "conversational" pace. Note that both approaches give you about the same amount of time at tempo.

The purpose of threshold work is to raise your lactate threshold. This occurs by improving your lactate tolerance and/or decreasing the amount of lactate accumulation in your blood. As you raise your lactate threshold, you are able to stay aerobic at faster speeds. See figure 5-4 for a summary of this type of workout; and see the swim, bike and run workouts at the end of the book for specific examples.

	Threshold Workout
When:	Late base training and beyond
Why:	To raise the lactate threshold by improving lactate tolerance and decreasing lactate accumulation, which allows the athlete to stay aerobic at faster speeds
What:	Sustained tempo for up to an hour or long intervals (e.g. 5-20 min) with a 5:1 work to recovery ratio. Intensity is at a "comfortably hard" pace, and can range from Zones 3-5a depending upon the point in the base-build-peak progression.
How:	Use heart rate, pace or perceived exertion to monitor intensity

Figure 5-4. Summary of the threshold workout

Doing these types of threshold workouts in Zone 3 acts as a stepping stone to work done in Zone 4 (and into Zone 5a). The ultimate aim of threshold training is to target the lactate threshold (Zones 4-5a). Work done in Zone 3 is therefore limited in base training to prepare you physically and mentally for the transition to higher intensity threshold work.

Develop Your Base: Late Base Training Sample Schedules

As with early base training, late base training still involves your staple endurance sessions, including the weekly "long" workout. In addition, you should continue to include drills in your recovery and/or endurance workouts. But now you can begin to replace the alactics with the "comfortably hard" aerobic tempo (Zone 3) or threshold (Zone 4) workouts. Tables 5-4, 5-5, and 5-6 illustrate sample weekly schedules for the late stages of base training for athletes doing two, three, and four workouts per discipline per week, respectively.

Table 5-4. Sample late base training week with 2 workouts/discipline

Day	Discipline	Workout
Monday	SWIM	Recovery w/drills
Tuesday	BIKE	Recovery w/drills
Wednesday	RUN	Recovery w/drills
Thursday	--	
Friday	SWIM	Endurance w/tempo
Saturday	BIKE	Endurance w/tempo
Sunday	RUN	Endurance w/tempo

In table 5-4, this triathlete incorporates some tempo work into the single endurance session of the week. The athlete might start with 10-15 minutes in Zone 3, or the lower end of "comfortably hard" pace. Alternatively, the athlete could perhaps start with 2 x 5-minute cruise intervals with 1-minute recovery interval in between. The athlete would then progress from there by first adding time at tempo and then upping the tempo into Zone 4 (the higher end of "comfortably hard" pace). The same strategy can be seen table 5-5 and table 5-6.

In sum, base training focuses on building your aerobic foundation and preparing the body for higher intensity work to be done down the road—namely, through the use of alactics (early to late stages) and tempo/threshold work (late stages). As you move through your base training, your training volume increases. This means the length of individual sessions increases—particularly the weekly long workout in each discipline—resulting in a gradual increase in weekly volume.

Keep in mind that the duration of each workout—along with the number of cruise intervals or time at tempo—should be based on your current level of fitness, where you are in your individual training progression, and the length of the race you are targeting. Begin where you currently are and progress gradually and systematically from there. Once you have built your base; then you will be ready to move into the next training phase and build upon that base.

Table 5-5. Sample late base training week with 3 workouts/discipline

Day	Discipline	Workout
Monday	--	
Tuesday	SWIM	Endurance w/tempo
	BIKE	Endurance w/tempo
Wednesday	SWIM	Recovery w/drills
	RUN	Endurance w/tempo
Thursday	BIKE/RUN	Recovery w/drills
Friday	SWIM	Long
Saturday	BIKE	Long
Sunday	RUN	Long

Table 5-6. Sample late base training week with 4 workouts/discipline

Day	Discipline	Workout
Monday	SWIM	Recovery w/drills
Tuesday	SWIM	Endurance w/tempo
	BIKE	Endurance w/tempo
Wednesday	BIKE/RUN	Endurance
	SWIM	Endurance
Thursday	RUN	Endurance w/tempo
	BIKE	Recovery w/drills
Friday	SWIM	Long
	RUN	Recovery w/drills
Saturday	BIKE	Long
Sunday	RUN	Long

Building Upon Your Base

Whereas base training primarily involves an increase in training volume, the build training phase is marked by a levelling off or reduction in volume with an increase in intensity. But keep in mind that regardless of the training phase, the bulk of your total training time will be done in the aerobic range.

In other words, during the build training phase time spent in Zones 1-2 still forms the largest portion of the training pie. But now you will dedicate some slices of that pie to higher intensity aerobic and anaerobic work. This means you will target threshold workouts done in Zones 4-5a, or "comfortably hard" pace. In addition, you will add VO_2max workouts in Zone 5b, or "uncomfortably hard" pace. More advanced and competitive triathletes, especially those targeting short course races, may add anaerobic capacity workouts in Zone 5c to the mix.

Threshold workouts have already been discussed (see again figure 5-4). You already began to incorporate these types of workouts during your late base training, whether at the low-level sub-threshold (Zone 3) or high-level sub-threshold (Zone 4). Now, you will continue to build upon your threshold work by targeting tempo and cruise intervals in Zones 4-5a and increasing the time spent near threshold. You also have two types of anaerobic workouts to draw from, discussed below.

VO$_2$max Workouts

The purpose of the VO$_2$max workouts is to increase the maximal rate of oxygen transport in your body (that is, your "aerobic capacity" or "VO$_2$max"), to build lactate tolerance (remember, lactate builds up at higher intensities), and to increase your anaerobic endurance. Ultimately, these workouts aim to help you learn *to be comfortable being uncomfortable*, which is what you need to do if you want to swim, bike and run as fast as you can over your race distance.

The VO$_2$max workouts consist of work intervals of 3 to 7 minutes in duration with a recovery interval equal to or slightly less than the work interval—for example, 3-minute work intervals with a 2-minute recovery interval in between. The intensity is in Zone 5b, or at "uncomfortably hard" pace. See figure 5-5 for a summary of this type of workout; and see the swim, bike and run workouts at the end of the book for specific examples.

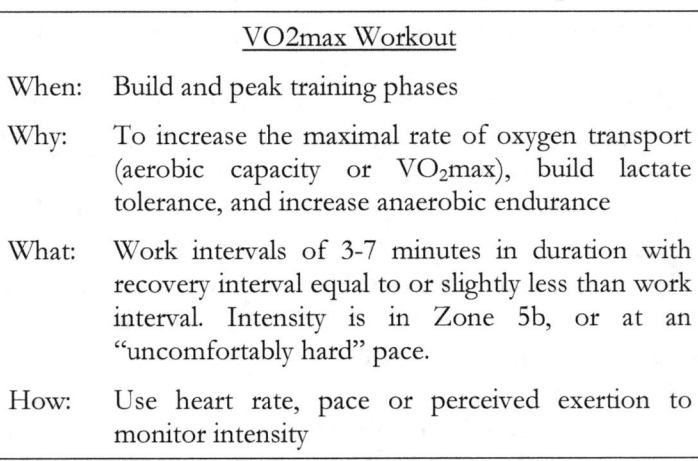

	VO2max Workout
When:	Build and peak training phases
Why:	To increase the maximal rate of oxygen transport (aerobic capacity or VO$_2$max), build lactate tolerance, and increase anaerobic endurance
What:	Work intervals of 3-7 minutes in duration with recovery interval equal to or slightly less than work interval. Intensity is in Zone 5b, or at an "uncomfortably hard" pace.
How:	Use heart rate, pace or perceived exertion to monitor intensity

Figure 5-5. Summary of the VO$_2$max workout

VO$_2$max workouts form a valuable addition to any triathlete's repertoire regardless of the distance you are racing. Even if you are racing long course events where you rarely venture into anaerobic territory, this type of anaerobic workout will help you perform better as an endurance athlete because, as noted earlier, it helps to expand your aerobic capacity. So don't shy away from VO$_2$max intervals. But do keep in mind that workouts in the anaerobic range take more out of you. They therefore require more recovery time. With anaerobic training, the saying that "a little goes a long way" holds true. And with all that said, you can still go far to improving your fitness and race times by simply focusing on threshold work even if you don't venture into higher end anaerobic training.

Anaerobic Capacity Workouts

The purpose of anaerobic capacity workouts is to improve your endurance in the anaerobic range, or your ability to maintain short durations of speed up to 2 minutes in duration. This is important for race starts, surges during a race where you need to match a competitor or drop a competitor, and finishing kicks.

	Anaerobic Capacity Workout
When:	Build and peak training phases
Why:	To improve the ability to maintain short durations of speed of up to 2 minutes in duration (starts, race surges, finishing kicks)
What:	Work intervals up to 2 minutes in duration with recovery interval equal to or greater than work interval to allow full recovery. Intensity is in Zone 5c, or at an "all out" pace.
How:	Use heart rate, pace or perceived exertion to monitor intensity

Figure 5-6. Summary of the anaerobic capacity workout

Anaerobic capacity workouts consist of work intervals up to 2 minutes in duration with a recovery interval equal to or greater than your work interval—for example, 1-minute work intervals with a 2-minute recovery interval in between. With these types of intervals, you want to recover fully in between each work bout. The intensity is in Zone 5c, or "all out" effort. See figure 5-6 for a summary of this type of workout; and see the swim, bike and run workouts at the end of the book for specific examples.

Build Upon Your Base: Build Phase Sample Schedules

Tables 5-7, 5-8, and 5-9 illustrate sample weekly schedules for the build training phase for athletes doing two, three, and four workouts per discipline per week, respectively. Common among these schedules is one or more endurance/recovery workouts plus a higher intensity workout. At first, that higher intensity workout targets threshold work. As you progress, that higher intensity workout targets VO_2max intervals. Eventually, anaerobic capacity intervals may also be added to the schedule, depending upon the goals and background of the athlete.

Aim to repeat a particular type of workout 5 to 12 times before progressing to a workout type of higher intensity; this will allow you to achieve the fitness gain from that type of workout and ensure you are ready to progress to the next level. This means you should do 5 to 12 threshold workouts for a given discipline before moving into VO_2max work for that discipline. Again, you can go far by simply focusing on threshold work. Don't skip or cut short your threshold work to prematurely jump into high intensity anaerobic work. Although you can reap great gains from VO_2max work, if you jump into it without an adequate base you risk greater exposure to injury and overtraining.

The approach of doing one higher intensity workout per discipline per week works well for most triathletes. However, advanced triathletes with a solid base can handle a threshold workout plus a VO_2max workout in later build or peak phases. You could also just single out one or two disciplines for a VO_2max workout in addition to a threshold workout in all three. This would allow you to target a discipline you need to improve the most.

Table 5-7. Sample build week with 2 workouts/discipline

Day	Discipline	Workout
Monday	SWIM	Recovery w/drills
Tuesday	BIKE	Threshold or VO$_2$max
Wednesday	RUN	Recovery w/drills
Thursday	SWIM	Threshold or VO$_2$max
Friday	BIKE	Recovery w/drills
Saturday	RUN	Threshold or VO$_2$max
Sunday	--	

Table 5-8. Sample build week with 3 workouts/discipline

Day	Discipline	Workout
Monday	--	
Tuesday	SWIM	Threshold or VO$_2$max
	BIKE	Threshold or VO$_2$max
Wednesday	SWIM	Recovery w/drills
	RUN	Recovery w/drills
Thursday	RUN	Threshold or VO$_2$max
	BIKE	Recovery w/drills
Friday	SWIM	Long
Saturday	BIKE	Long
Sunday	RUN	Long

Keep in mind that anaerobic work for swimming, and even cycling, will take less of a toll on the body than anaerobic work for running. Doing your VO$_2$max run workouts on an incline and/or on more forgiving surfaces (e.g. grass, dirt) will lessen the strain on your body's supporting structures.

In sum, building upon your base involves gradually adding higher intensity work on top of your aerobic foundation. This involves work directly above/below your lactate threshold and anaerobic work. To successfully handle the increase in intensity, reduce the total weekly volume in your schedule. Given that "a little intensity goes a long way" and the fact that "all intensity all the time" is a recipe for overtraining, keep in mind that the bulk of your training time during the build phase remains dedicated to aerobic work in Zones 1-2. This allows you to actively recover in between the interval sessions and to continue to add to your aerobic foundation. As always, begin where you currently are and progress gradually and systematically from there. Once you have built your base and built upon that base; then you are ready to peak for your target race.

Table 5-9. Sample build week with 4 workouts/discipline

Day	Discipline	Workout
Monday	SWIM	Recovery w/drills
Tuesday	SWIM	Threshold or VO_2max
	BIKE	Threshold or VO_2max
Wednesday	BIKE/RUN	Endurance
	SWIM	Endurance
Thursday	RUN	Threshold or VO_2max
	BIKE	Recovery w/drills
Friday	SWIM	Long
	RUN	Recovery w/drills
Saturday	BIKE	Long
Sunday	RUN	Long

Peaking for Your Target Race

In the art and science of triathlon training, peaking for your top priority event is certainly as much an art as a science. Different athletes respond in different ways to the final taper; and this is where experience and knowing yourself will allow you to craft an effective training schedule over the final weeks before your target race. Nevertheless, there are certain principles that you need to keep in mind during your peak training phase.

The peak phase covers the last few or more weeks before your target race. The general focus consists of decreasing volume while maintaining or increasing intensity. The aim here is to sharpen and hone your fitness. The foundation of the house has been laid, and the fixtures have been put in place; now you just need polish the fixtures to make the house shine.

There are two common errors athletes often make when peaking for an event. Some athletes mistake the notion of "tapering" for simply taking time off to rest. Although rest is vital during this (and any) phase, remember that the vacation doesn't start until after your race. For these athletes, too much time off and too little intensity leaves them feeling stale as they toe the starting line.

Other athletes get nervous about the reduction of volume during their taper and feel they need to do more to stay fit and be ready for race day. These are the ones that sneak in extra intervals or extra workouts. As a result, they do too much and reach the starting line feeling overly fatigued. Although maintaining some volume and intensity throughout peak training is essential, remember that your fitness is already in the bank. This isn't the time to continue making large deposits; it's time to begin the withdrawals to buy the freshness and sharpness required for peak performance.

Avoiding these two extremes requires balancing your reduction of volume with your use of intensity. To avoid the problem of too many days off, keep the same frequency of workouts throughout the week; but simply reduce the duration of those workouts. This reduces the overall volume while allowing you to maintain your familiar routine.

When implementing intensity, reduce the number of intervals you do. Again, this reduces volume. You should leave the workout feeling less fatigued; and should feel yourself getting fresher and more eager to race as the days go on. This surplus of energy can be difficult to harness for some. The temptation is to do more intervals or go harder during a planned tempo or recovery workout. But this is where you need to reign yourself in and save it for the race. Trust in your training and trust in your plan. You will have time to fully test your mettle come race day.

Peak for Your Race: Peak Phase Sample Schedules

Tables 5-10, 5-11, and 5-12 illustrate sample weekly schedules during the peak training phase for athletes doing two, three, and four workouts per discipline per week, respectively.

Table 5-10. Sample peak training week with 2 workouts/discipline

Day	Discipline	Workout
Monday	SWIM	Recovery w/drills
Tuesday	BIKE	VO$_2$max
Wednesday	RUN	Recovery w/drills
Thursday	SWIM	VO$_2$max
Friday	BIKE	Recovery w/drills
Saturday	RUN	VO$_2$max
Sunday	--	

For the triathlete in table 5-10, the schedule looks similar to the one used during the build phase. Here, however, the athlete would reduce the duration of each workout. On the days marked by intensity—namely, VO$_2$max—the number of intervals would be reduced over what the athlete had previously been doing during the build phase.

The triathlete in table 5-11, also maintains the same number of workouts per discipline per week. However, some of the workouts (now shortened) have been combined to more closely simulate race conditions. See, for example, the bike/run brick workout on Tuesday that features VO$_2$max intervals. A short dose of intensity on Tuesday is then followed by two easy days to allow the legs to fully recover before a second bike/run brick on Friday. Intensity punctuated by a few days of recovery is the general pattern. Likewise, for the triathlete in table 5-12, the schedule has been changed to balance more recovery with the intensity.

If you are doing multiple races at the end of the season, you can reasonably expect to maintain peak form for up to three to four weeks but not much longer. In between the races, aim for a race intensity workout every three to four days with ample short, recovery workouts to stay loose and fresh.

Table 5-11. Sample peak training week with 3 workouts/discipline

Day	Discipline	Workout
Monday	SWIM	VO_2max
Tuesday	BIKE/RUN	VO_2max
Wednesday	RUN	Recovery w/alactics
Thursday	SWIM	VO_2max
Friday	BIKE/RUN	VO_2max
	SWIM	Recovery w/alactics
Saturday	BIKE	Recovery w/alactics
Sunday	--	

Table 5-12. Sample peak training week with 4 workouts/discipline

Day	Discipline	Workout
Monday	SWIM	VO_2max
Tuesday	BIKE/RUN	VO_2max
	SWIM	Recovery
Wednesday	RUN	Recovery w/alactics
Thursday	SWIM	VO_2max
	BIKE	Recovery
Friday	BIKE/RUN	VO_2max
	SWIM	Recovery w/alactics
Saturday	BIKE	Recovery w/alactics
	RUN	Recovery
Sunday	--	

Race Week

In the final week before your target race, your mantra should be "sharpen, hone, and rest." I typically schedule a day off two days prior to the event. It takes about two days for the body to catch up with what you do—whether in terms of rest or a workout. So if you hammer intervals two days before your race, your body will feel the maximum effect of those intervals (in terms of fatigue) on race day. Likewise, if you rest two days before your race, your body will reap the maximum rewards of that rest on race day. The same goes for a good night's sleep and a good dinner. Focus on the night of sleep and dinner two days before your race.

Then, use the day before your race to do a short warmup in each discipline. This loosens you up and shakes off any cobwebs from the day off so that you are ready to go come race morning. These warmup workouts also give you an opportunity to do a final equipment check and potentially to run through the transitions if they are open. Avoid the temptation to "race" those workouts. You may have lots of energy and be eager to race. But remember, these should be easy warmups with a few alactics to get the muscles moving and heart rate firing a bit. Given the excitement that often surrounds the pre-race day expo, you might be better off doing your workouts away from the race site. Also, this probably isn't the best time to hook up with new training partners unless you are adamant about following your own pace and achieving what you need to accomplish in those pre-race day workouts (rather than getting caught up in an overly competitive "warmup" the day before the actual race).

Race Day Warmup

You've put in the training and now you're ready to toe the starting line for your race. But one last question remains in your mind: how long should my warmup be? This question rightly assumes that some sort of warmup will be important to get the most out of your race.

The warmup plays an important role in injury prevention and

readies the body for the rigors of race level intensity. Cold muscles are tight muscles; and tight muscles are more susceptible to strains and tears. A warmup raises the temperature of working muscles. It leads to vasodilation, or the widening of blood vessels, which increases blood flow throughout the body. This also sends more oxygen to working muscles to produce energy to fuel your activity. The speed of nerve transmissions increases, along with the speed and force of muscle contractions. And joint mobility and flexibility are enhanced. In short, a proper warmup prepares the body to handle race level intensity from the time the starting gun fires.

As a general rule of thumb, the length of your warmup is inversely proportional to the length of the race. The shorter the race, the longer the warmup should be. In shorter races (or even in longer distance races for elites), the intensity from the start will be high. To be able to match that intensity from the gun, the engine needs to be fully revved up so it can fire on all cylinders. This requires a warmup that starts early and includes some higher intensity activity to raise the heart rate and get the muscles firing at race pace and faster.

In contrast, the longer the race, the shorter the warmup needs to be. In longer races (or even in shorter races for novice athletes), the racing distance tends to exceed a day's typical training mileage. As a result, the intensity from the start is not as great. At these distances, the athlete can use the beginning part of the race as an extension of the shorter warmup begun prior to the starting gun. This especially applies to long course racers who need a pre-race routine that provides a light warmup while conserving energy and muscle glycogen for the long effort ahead.

Regardless of the distance to be raced, there are many pre-race logistics that also take up one's time on race morning. With this in mind, it is a good idea to arrive 60 to 90 minutes prior to the start. Even if you already picked up your bib and timing chip the day before, you will need time on race morning to get your body marked, set up your transition area, and orient to the flow of traffic through T1 and T2 (not to mention find an available port-a-potty). Also keep in mind that in many races the transition area closes a certain amount of time before the first wave starts—which may or may not be your wave. So plan accordingly and give yourself time to get organized before you have to leave the transition area.

Once you have claimed your spot in the transition area, start your warmup with a few minutes of neuromuscular activation followed by about 5 minutes of dynamic stretching. See the Alp Fitness website (alpfitness.com) for video demos of warmup activities. From there, move into the cardiovascular component. For sprint and Olympic distance races, it's good to touch base with all three disciplines. I prefer to do them in reverse order, starting with 10 to 15 minutes of running, followed by 10 to 15 minutes of cycling, and ending with 10 to 15 minutes of swimming. Others may prefer a bike-run order before heading to the water for some swimming. Still others may prefer to simply bike and swim, or to run and swim.

Although the run portion of the race is the farthest off, running still forms an important part of the pre-race warmup. Running is very effective and efficient at elevating the heart rate and producing a light sweat—two general objectives you want to achieve during the warmup. Even if you only do a few minutes, it's also a good confidence booster to know that your running muscles are firing and ready to go. And if you are unable to bike or swim due to logistical issues (such as a closed swim course or not being able to take your bike out of the transition area), running will be an indispensable warmup activity.

For shorter races, biking should also be part of the warmup. Depending upon personal preference, this can be done before or after you run. After some easy spinning at warmup pace, include a few surges to elevate your heart rate to race pace. At bigger or more crowded races, it may be difficult (or simply not allowed) to take your bike out of the transition area once you check in. In that case, you might want to bring a stationary trainer. Remember to always wear your helmet with chinstrap buckled while on your bike (even on a stationary trainer). USA Triathlon rules apply during the warmup, and you don't want to get disqualified before the race even starts.

Given that the race starts with the swim, it is best to do the swim portion of your warmup last. After 5 to 10 minutes of swimming at warmup pace, include some short sprints with ample recovery plus a few minutes of tempo swimming at race pace. The aim is to elevate your heart rate into the zones you will be using at the start of the race and during the swim. This will prime you for the action once the gun goes off.

At some races, be aware that you might not be able to get into the water before the start—either due to course restrictions or cold water temperatures that make it counterproductive to warming up. In those cases, you will need to adapt by relying on running and/or cycling to raise your heart rate and work up a light sweat before going to the starting line.

Table 5-13. Pre-race warmup protocol for short course triathlons

Time	Activity
90 minutes prior	Arrive, check-in, set up transition area, use toilet
70 minutes prior	3-5 minutes muscle activation exercises
65 minutes prior	3-5 minutes dynamic stretching, leg swings
60 minutes prior	10-15 minutes running at warmup pace with 2-4 strides of 15-30 seconds
45 minutes prior	10-15 minutes biking at warmup pace with 2-4 surges of 15-30 seconds
30 minutes prior	Final check of transition area, put on wetsuit, head to water
25 minutes prior	10-15 minutes swimming at warmup pace with 2-4 surges of 15-30 seconds
5 minutes prior	Line up for start

The specific shape your warmup takes will depend on how hard you plan on racing, how well you are conditioned for the distance, and the length of the race. If you are a highly competitive swimmer looking to get out front at the start; then your swim warmup needs to be tailored accordingly. On the other hand, if you are a novice swimmer looking to simply stay out of the fray with a fairly calm, low intensity swim; then use your swim warmup to acclimate to the water.

But regardless of your race goals or race distance, you will benefit from some sort of warmup that readies the body for the race. The key is to find a routine that works for you; then ritualize that routine so you can move through the checklist on auto-pilot. Table 5-13 provides a sample warmup protocol for short course triathlons, and table 5-14 provides a sample warmup schedule for long course triathlons.

Table 5-14. Pre-race warmup protocol for long course triathlons

Time	Activity
90 minutes prior	Arrive, check-in, set up transition area, use toilet
50 minutes prior	3-5 minutes muscle activation exercises
45 minutes prior	3-5 minutes dynamic stretching, leg swings
40 minutes prior	5-10 minutes running (or cycling) at warmup pace (less for Ironman)
30 minutes prior	Final check of transition area, put on wetsuit, head to water
25 minutes prior	10-15 minutes swimming at warmup pace with 2-4 surges of 15-30 seconds
5 minutes prior	Line up for start

Summary of Base-Build-Peak Progression

To summarize, base training develops your aerobic foundation as you gradually increase your training volume. The bulk of your training is done in the lower aerobic zones. To that, you add alactics, drills, and functional strength training (the topic of the next chapter). As you progress in your base training, add higher intensity aerobic tempo, or sub-threshold work.

As you move into the build training phase, volume levels off or decreases while you focus on increasing intensity in the form of threshold and anaerobic workouts.

The peak training phase covers the last several weeks prior to your target race. Here, you maintain frequency of training while reducing the duration of those workouts. The aim is to sharpen and hone your race readiness through a balance of intensity and recovery. Figure 5-7 summarizes the base-build-peak progression.

Establish and Develop Your Base

In early stages, start with:
- Endurance workouts
- Recovery workouts
- Include alactics
- Include drills

In late stages, add:
- Aerobic tempo workouts
- Threshold workouts

Build Upon Your Base

Add to the endurance workouts:
- Threshold workouts
- VO_2max workouts
- Anaerobic capacity workouts

Peak for Your Race

Volume:
- Maintain frequency of workouts
- Reduce duration of workouts

Intensity:
- Maintain or increase intensity
- Reduce number of intervals

Rest and recovery:
- Recovery workouts
- Extra sleep/rest

Figure 5-7. Summary of the base-build-peak progression

Part III

Supplemental Training

6
FUNCTIONAL STRENGTH

Functional strength work is an essential element of your training to help you become stronger, more efficient and less injury prone. Although the principle of specificity states that you must dedicate a substantial amount of training time to the activities in which you will compete, spending all your training time simply swimming, cycling and running is a recipe for overuse injuries. This is where supplemental strength training becomes an indispensable tool in the triathlete's repertoire. Functional work can target muscular imbalances to provide the supporting structure needed to excel in your events. Functional work is as much about making your muscles "smarter" as making them stronger so you move more effectively and efficiently.

Building "Smarter" and Stronger Muscles

When most people think of strength training, they think of making their muscles stronger. But strong muscles aren't worth much if they don't fire when needed or coordinate with each other during sport specific movements. For endurance athletes engaged in strength training, it is important to recognize that stronger muscles form only part of the equation for enhanced performance. You also need to have good neuromuscular control over those muscles.

Any time a muscle contracts, it requires a signal from the nervous system. This is why we talk about neuromuscular movement (as opposed to just muscular movement). A great deal of the work done by the nervous system occurs more or less automatically as a result of patterns set down over time. We call this "muscle memory."

If you play the guitar, your fingers seem to "know" where to go to play a C chord, for example, without consciously placing them on the strings. Of course, it takes a while to build up mastery of those movement patterns. In general, it takes about 4,000 to 6,000 repetitions to change or develop new muscle memory patterns.

As athletes, the movements we make are built up over time in the same way. Poor form—and resulting injuries—can be a result of weak muscles, inhibition of muscles needed for a movement, or a combination of weak muscles that don't fire when needed. Functional strength work targets typical areas of muscular imbalances while teaching you to use those muscles in ways that carry over into your sport specific activities.

So to say we want to make our muscles "smart" as well as strong means that we're aiming to develop neuromuscular control in addition to strength. This is why it is always essential to perform the exercises—as well as your endurance sports (running, swimming, cycling)—with proper form. You want to ingrain positive habits into your muscle memory.

Endurance athletes are eager to find ways to improve their performance, and many embrace strength training. Yet some of those who embrace strength training view it from a one sided perspective. For them, it is all about making muscles stronger without regard to function. If strength training doesn't involve heavy weights that target isolated muscle groups (e.g. machine weights); then they don't feel like they're getting a "good workout." Likewise, they see suggestions to incorporate supplemental functional work into daily activities in short spurts of a few minutes as too little or inconsequential to constitute a "good workout." For them, it is easy to blow off that daily 10 minute functional strength session.

But if you shift your perspective on functional strength training to take in the broader picture of what you're trying to accomplish—stronger and smarter muscles—then it is easier to see the benefit of the supplemental work.

Let's return to the analogy of learning to play the guitar.

Imagine this scenario. Let's say you show up for your two hour guitar lesson once a week without picking up the guitar in between those weekly sessions. It takes the first part of the lesson to remember what you've forgotten over the past week. And by the end of the session, brain fatigue sets in and limits your ability to effectively practice the assigned chords. But you definitely walk away from the session feeling like you got the equivalent of a "good workout." Your fingers hurt, you're tired, etc.

Now image this scenario. You still dedicate 2 hours a week to practicing your guitar, but now your weekly lesson takes 1 hour and you spend 10 minutes each day in between the weekly lessons practicing the movement patterns for the chords assigned that week. In each of those 10-minute daily sessions, you may not feel like you're getting the equivalent of a "good workout," but you gradually begin to learn the chords. And you do so sooner than in the first scenario.

Contrasting these two scenarios underscores the point that making your muscles smarter benefits from consistent, frequent reinforcement of the neuromuscular patterns that contribute to muscle memory. If it takes 4,000 to 6,000 repetitions to ingrain movement patterns into muscle memory, it is best to spread those repetitions out in short but frequent sessions rather than lumping them all together in longer but infrequent sessions.

The bottom line? Don't think it is inconsequential to incorporate short but frequent functional strength sessions or neuromuscular drills into your daily activities. Step away from the desk during the workday to do a few minutes of planks or donkey kicks or balance drills, for example.

It may seem like nothing when you are training up to 8, 12, 15 or more hours a week in multisport endurance activities. But attention to this supplemental work will help you reinforce movement patterns needed for good neuromuscular control.

When it comes to optimal performance come race day, your muscles need to be more than strong. They also need to be smart.

Individual Exercises

The rest of this chapter features several functional strength exercises for triathletes. Access video demos on the Alp Fitness website (alpfitness.com). Keep in mind that time-crunched athletes need only dedicate an extra 10 minutes a day to make a difference. If you can't spare any extra time before or after your swimming, cycling or running sessions, then consider squeezing in that 10 minutes before breakfast in the morning (a great way to start the day and get the blood flowing), while taking a break from work in the afternoon (a great way to alleviate the stress of sitting at a desk), or while watching your favorite television show in the evening (use the commercials as training intervals).

Good Mornings

Start with feet shoulder width apart. Put your shoulder blades "in your back pockets" so you are standing tall.

Keeping your back flat with knees slightly bent, push your hips backwards to "hinge" from the hips. Keep your weight over your heels and eyes looking forward (not downward). Bend as far as your range of motion allows with a straight back (stop if your back starts to round). Squeeze the glutes and return to a standing position.

You want to primarily feel the glutes working (rather than the lower back). If you are feeling your lower back working, focus on squeezing the glutes to shift the workload to the butt.

Perform 1-5 sets of 8-12 reps per leg. Or, perform 1-5 sets of 20-40 second intervals (doing as many reps as possible during those intervals).

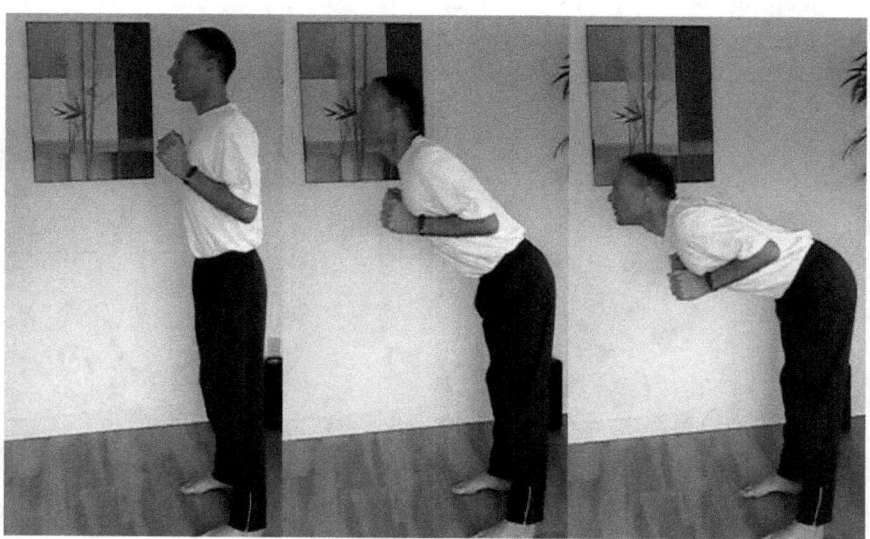

Figure 6-1. Good mornings

Superman

Start in the prone position (lying face down). Lift your left arm and right leg off the ground. As you place your left arm and right leg back on the ground, raise your right arm and left leg off the ground. Alternate this motion for time (e.g. 20-30 seconds) or for a designated number of reps (e.g. 10-20).

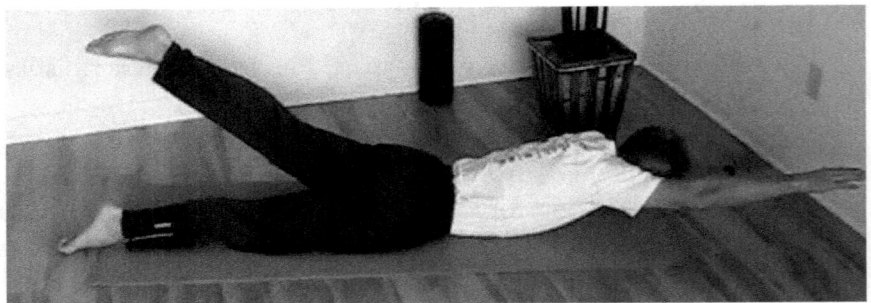

Figure 6-2. Superman

Back Extension

Start lying on the floor in the prone position (face down). Pull your elbows into the rib cage and lift upper body off the ground, leading with the chest. Squeeze the shoulder blades. Return upper body to the ground. Repeat for a designated time (e.g. 20-30 seconds) or number of reps (e.g. 8-12).

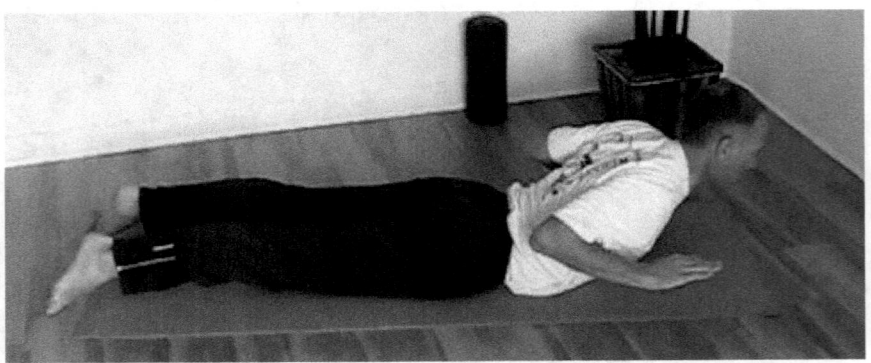

Figure 6-3. Back extension

Front Plank

Lie in prone position (face down). Place toes on ground in dorsiflexed position. Place elbows under shoulders. Squeeze the quads. Squeeze the glutes. And raise into a plank. Keep the back flat. Do not let the butt rise or sink. Stay flat. Hold for 30 seconds to 3 minutes, breaking up with rest as needed.

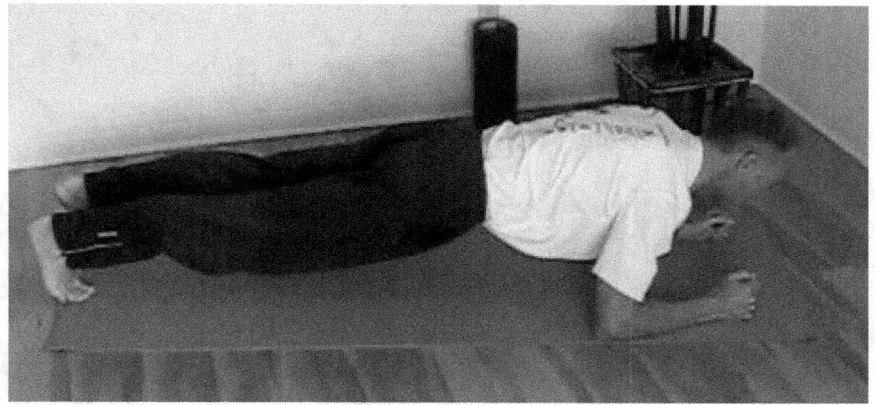

Figure 6-4. Front plank

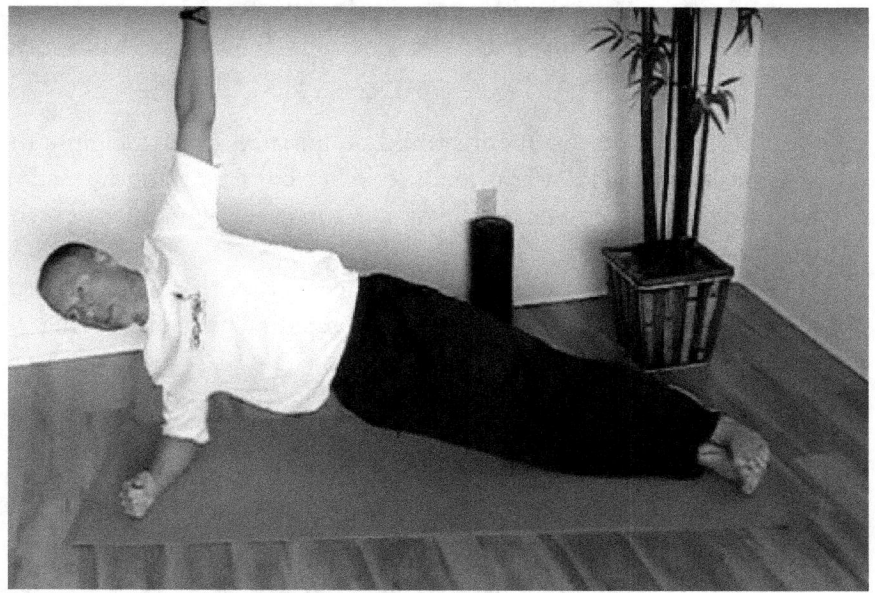

Figure 6-5. Side plank

Side Plank

Lie on side. Put top foot in front of bottom foot (easier) or stack top foot on top of bottom foot (harder). Push up into a side plank (use top hand if needed as a brace). Use hand as a brace (easiest). Move hand to hips (harder). Raise hand in air (hardest). Hold for 30 seconds to 3 minutes per side, breaking up with rest as needed.

Donkey Kicks

Get on the floor on hands and knees. Keep back straight as with the plank. Keeping back flat and still, squeeze the glute to move one leg back and slightly to the side (like a donkey kicking).

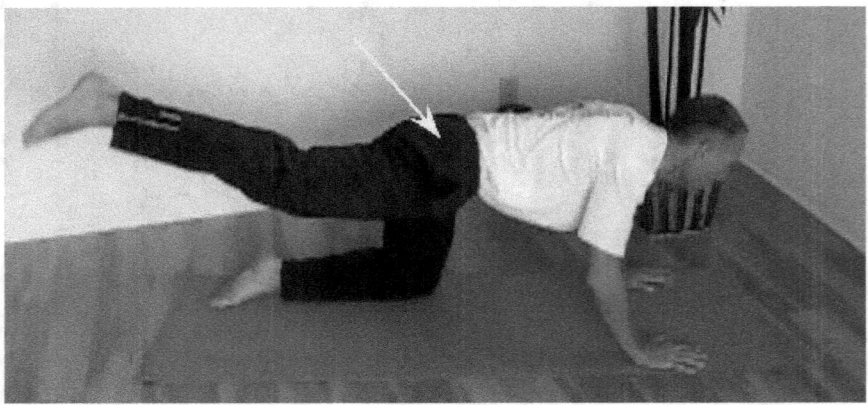

Figure 6-6. Donkey kicks

Note that the movement should be initiated from the glute (butt), not the lower back. If you feel the lower back working instead, start with smaller movements until you can increase the range of extension using only the glute.

Perform 1-5 sets of 8-12 reps per leg. Or, perform 1-5 sets of 20-40 second intervals (doing as many reps as possible during those intervals).

Hip Abductions (Lying)

Lie on side. Stack top foot on top of bottom foot. Dorsiflex (bring toes to knee) and slightly pigeon toe top foot (this is the position to keep your foot in for the raises).

Squeeze medial glute (side of hip) to raise leg as high as you can. Lower leg back down in a controlled manner. Repeat.

Perform 1-5 sets of 8-12 reps per leg. Or, perform 1-5 sets of 20-40 second intervals (doing as many reps as possible during those intervals).

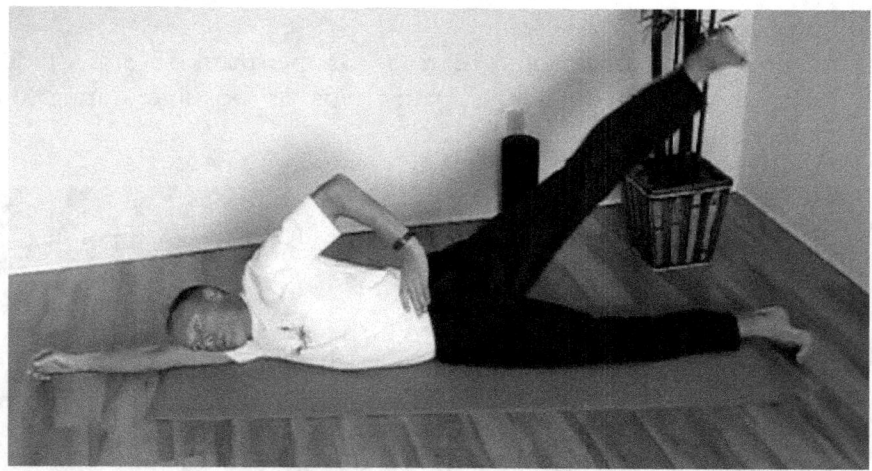

Figure 6-7. Lying leg raises, or hip abductions (a.k.a. Jane Fondas)

Hip Abductions (Standing)

These are a standing version of the lying hip abductions. The standing version engages more core muscles as you balance on one leg.

Stand on one foot. Maintain a tall and straight body position. Squeeze medial glute (side of hip) to abduct (move away from body) as far as you can. Return leg to midline in a controlled manner. Repeat.

Perform 1-5 sets of 8-12 reps per leg. Or, perform 1-5 sets of 20-40 second intervals (doing as many reps as possible during those intervals).

Squats

Start with feet shoulder width apart. Put your shoulder blades "in your back pockets" so you are standing tall.

Keeping your back flat, push your hips backwards as you bend slightly at the knees. Here, you are "hinging" from the hips as you go into a squat. Keep your weight over your heels.

As you squat (again, keeping the back flat and hinging from the hips), raise your arms out in front as a counter balance. Go to parallel or deeper as long as you can maintain the flat back.

Squeeze the glutes and return to a standing position.

The key is to initiate the movement by hinging at the hips with a flat back. You should feel your glutes working (not the quads). Done properly, this is a glute exercise!

Perform 1-5 sets of 8-12 reps. Or, perform 1-5 sets of 20-40 second intervals (doing as many reps as possible during those intervals).

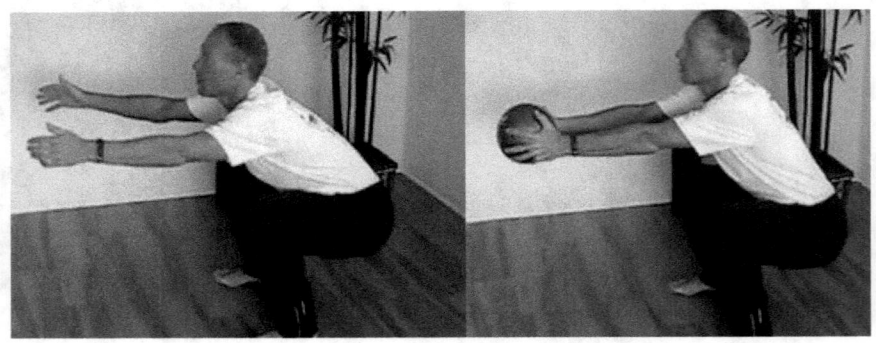

Figure 6-8. Body squat (left) and with medicine ball (right)

Squats (Single Leg)

Doing this in front of a mirror can be helpful to monitor form.

Start with a firm foundation on one leg (weight evenly distributed over forefoot and rear foot). Lift up the other leg. Pushing the hips backward (hinging from the hips), bend slight at the knee to go into a squat.

Go as far as you can without breaking form. Proper form means you move straight down and up (as in a double leg squat) without letting your knee or hips dive in or out and without losing balance or foot contact.

Think quality. Only perform as many single leg squats as you can with perfect form. Start with one and progress from there. Balance drills and hip/glute strengthening with other exercises will help improve your ability to do single leg squats.

Running is effectively a series of alternating single leg squats. Improve your coordination and strength here and you will become a better runner!

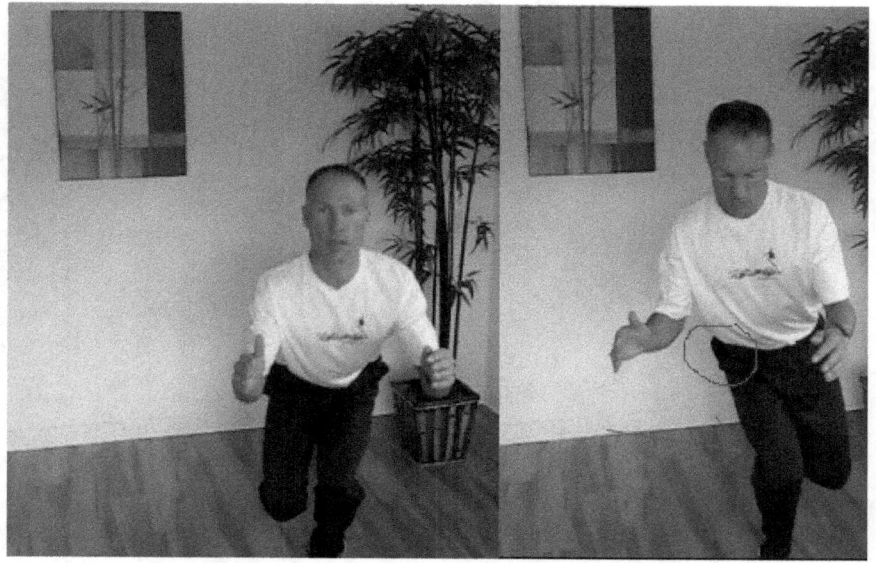

Figure 6-9. Single leg squat (left) and what to avoid (right)

Glute Bridge

Lie on back with knees bent. Squeeze glutes (butt) and raise up into a bridge. Return to ground in controlled manner.

Note that the muscles working should be the glutes (butt), not the quads (front of leg) or lower back. Be sure to initiate the movement by squeezing the glutes.

Perform 1-5 sets of 8-12 reps per leg. Or, perform 1-5 sets of 20-40 second intervals (doing as many reps as possible during those intervals).

Glute Bridge (Single Leg)

Lie on back with knees bent. Lift one leg up or place across opposite knee. Squeeze glute and raise up into a bridge. Return to ground in controlled manner.

Note that the muscle working should be the glute (butt), not the quads (front of leg) or lower back. Be sure to initiate the movement by squeezing the glute.

Perform 1-5 sets of 8-12 reps per leg. Or, perform 1-5 sets of 20-40 second intervals (doing as many reps as possible during those intervals).

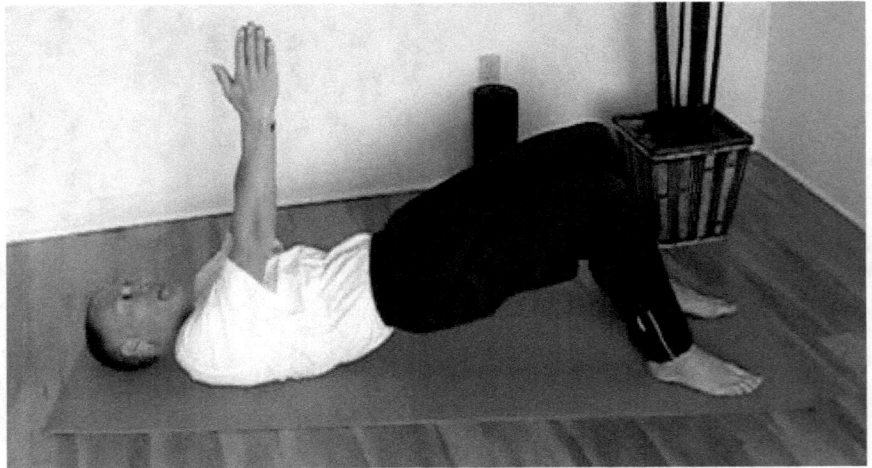

Figure 6-10. Glute bridge

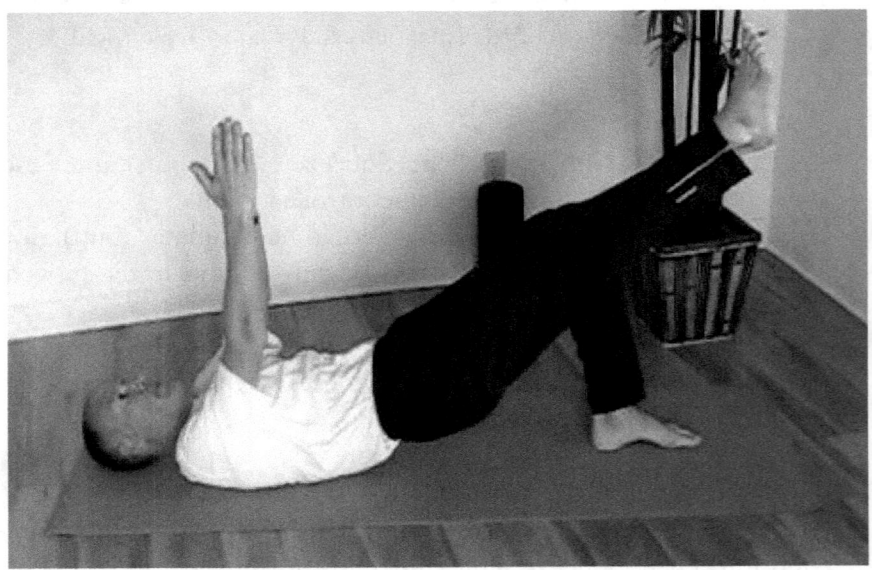

Figure 6-11. Single leg glute bridge

Front Plank with Straight Leg Hip Extension

This combines the front plank with straight leg hip extensions. In other words, you perform straight leg hip extensions from the front plank position. Alternatively, you can also perform a bent leg donkey kick from the plank position.

To get into the front plank position: Lie in prone position (face down). Place toes on ground in dorsiflexed position. Place elbows under shoulders. Squeeze the quads. Squeeze the glutes. And raise into a plank.

Keep the back flat. Do not let the butt rise or sink. Stay flat. Now, squeeze one glute to vertically raise that leg. Keep the back flat and still. Initiate and complete the movement from the glute.

If you feel the lower back or hamstring working, work on straight leg hip extensions while lying on the ground before progressing to the plank position. This should work the glute.

Perform 1-5 sets of 8-12 reps per leg. Or, perform 1-5 sets of 20-40 second intervals (doing as many reps as possible during those intervals).

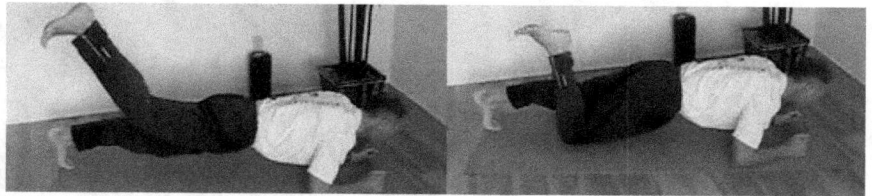

Figure 6-12. Front plank with straight leg (left) and bent leg (right) lift

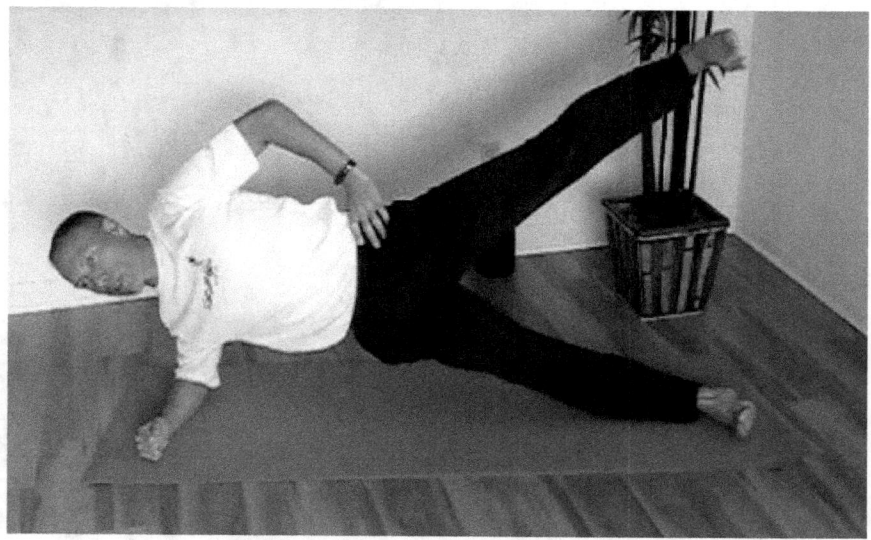

Figure 6-13. Side plank with hip abduction

Side Plank with Hip Abduction

This combines the side plank with lying hip abductions. In other words, you perform hip abductions (side leg raises) from the side plank position.

To get into the side plank position: Lie on side. Stack top foot on top of bottom foot. Push up into a side plank.

Now, squeeze the medial glute (side of hip) to raise leg as high as you can. Lower leg back down in a controlled manner. Repeat.

Perform 1-5 sets of 8-12 reps per leg. Or, perform 1-5 sets of 20-40 second intervals (doing as many reps as possible during those intervals).

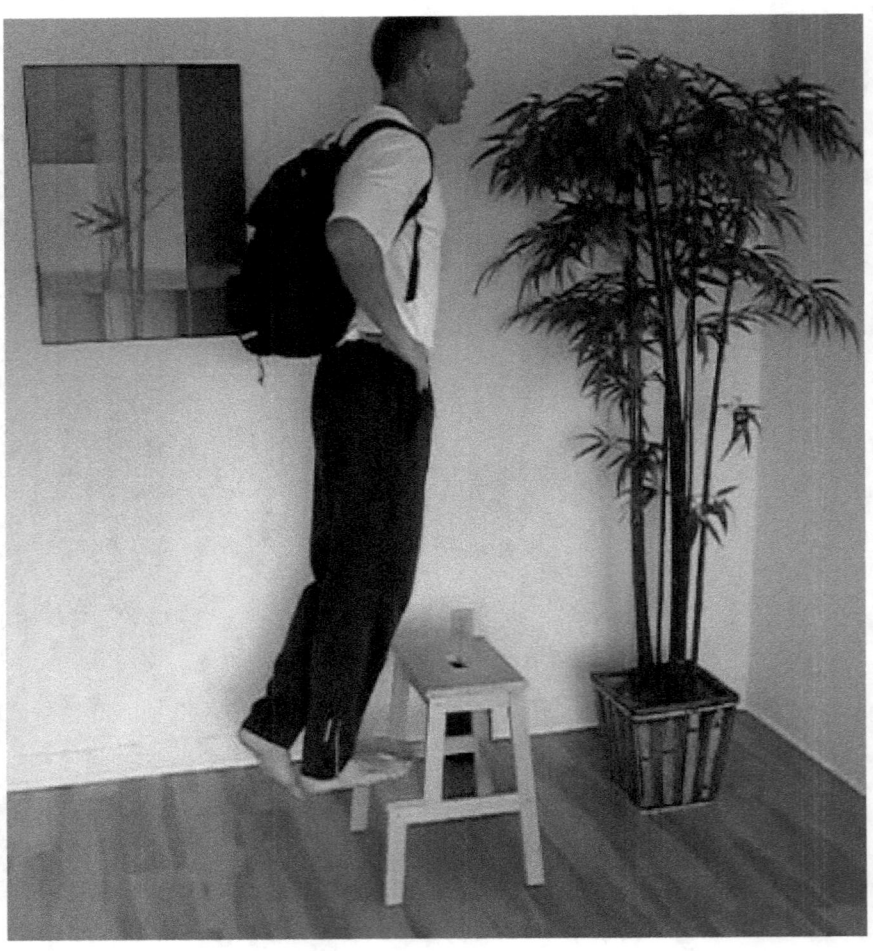

Figure 6-14. Eccentric calf raise

Eccentric Calf Raise

Raise up with both legs and down with one leg. 3 x 30 reps per leg per day. Week 1: body weight to flat. Week 2: body weight to drop (done on stair or slant board). Week 3-6: progressively add weight in a backpack up to 45-55 pounds. These are done daily for 6 weeks to repair chronic Achilles tendinopathy.

External Shoulder Rotation

This exercise targets the muscles involved in external rotation (infraspinatus and teres minor), which tend to be weak in swimmers. There are several variations of this exercise. But no matter which variation you do, start by squeezing your shoulder blades together and lowering them as if you were putting those shoulder blades in your back pockets. Maintain this posture throughout the exercise.

Variation #1. With a stretch cord in both hands, stand with arms at your side. To get into the starting position, bend your arms at your elbows to raise them to 90° in front of you. From this starting position, keep your elbows at your side (and keep your shoulder blades in your back pockets) as you rotate away from the midline of your body. This will pull the stretch cord apart. Slowly return to the starting position and repeat.

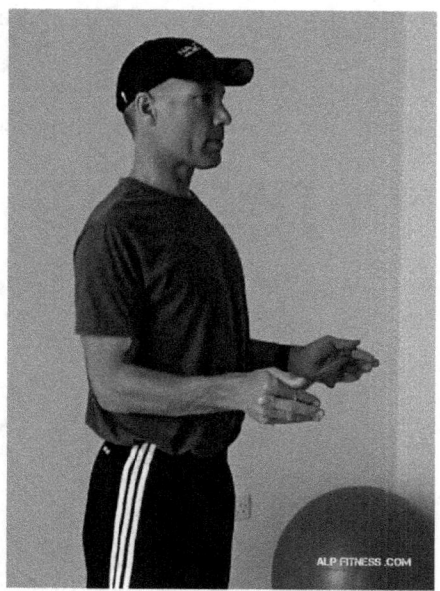

Figure 6-15. External rotation (starting point)

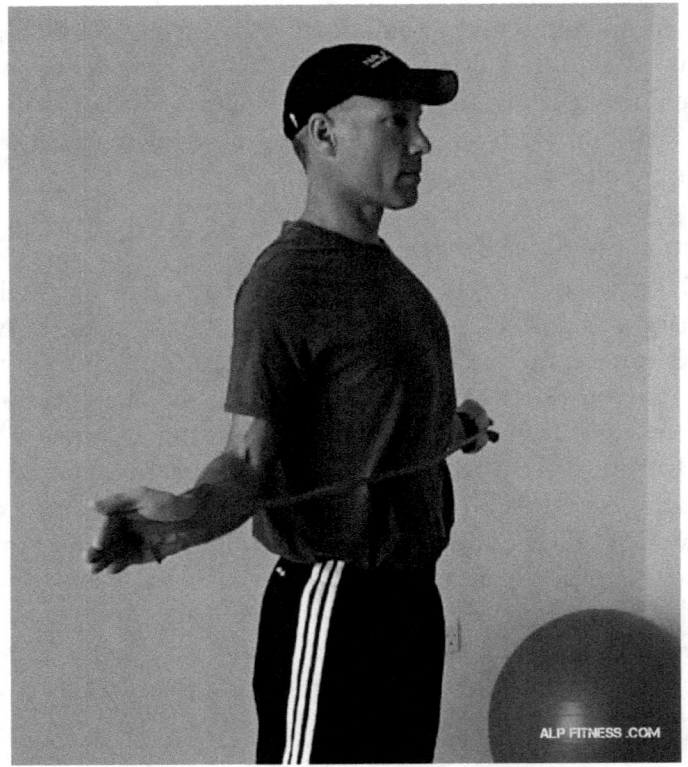

Figure 6-16. External rotation (ending point)

Variation #2. This is the same movement as in #1 but you do one arm at a time with the stretch cord affixed to a stable object.

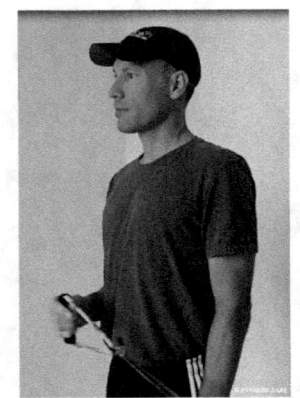

Figure 6-17. External rotation

Variation #3. Like #1 and #2, this also involves the same movement but that movement is done while lying on your side. Instead of a stretch cord, use a light weight as you externally rotate.

Variation #4. This variation is truly different than the first three in that you will perform external rotation with arms abducted to 90°. Get into the same starting position as in #1 and #2, but then raise your elbows so your upper arms are horizontal; this is your starting position. From here, externally rotate so that your arms will move from a horizontal position (pointing forward) to a vertical position (pointing to the sky). Remember to squeeze your shoulder blades and keep them in that position while doing the exercise. Slowly return and repeat. Try this without weight at first; as you progress you can add a light weight or resistance with a stretch cord.

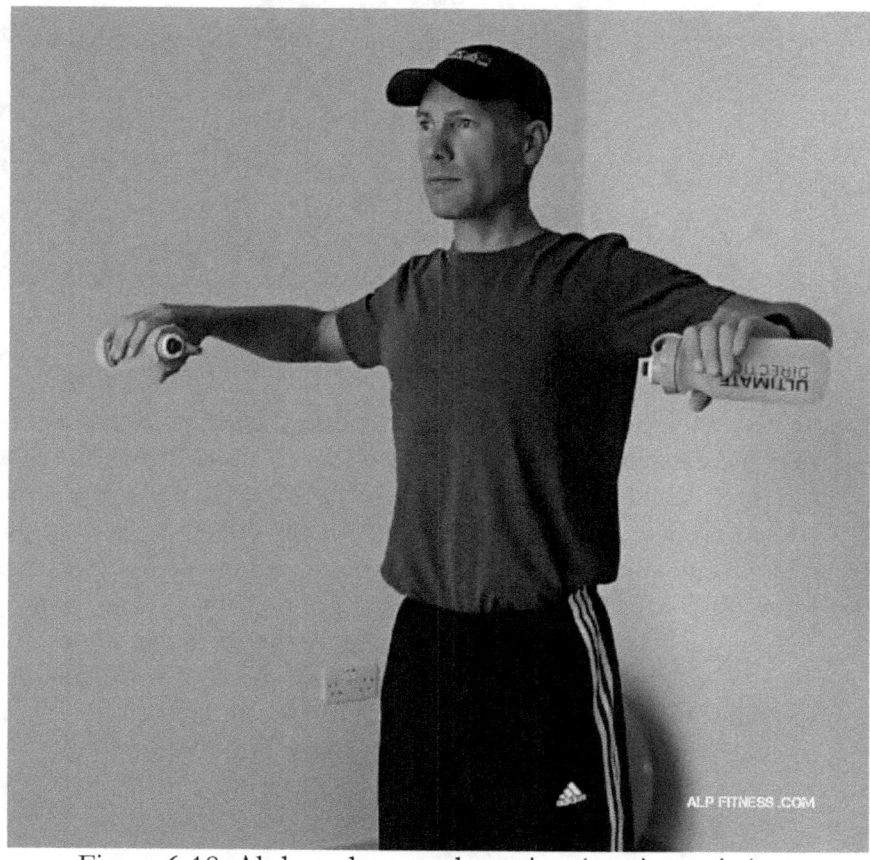

Figure 6-18. Abducted external rotation (starting point)

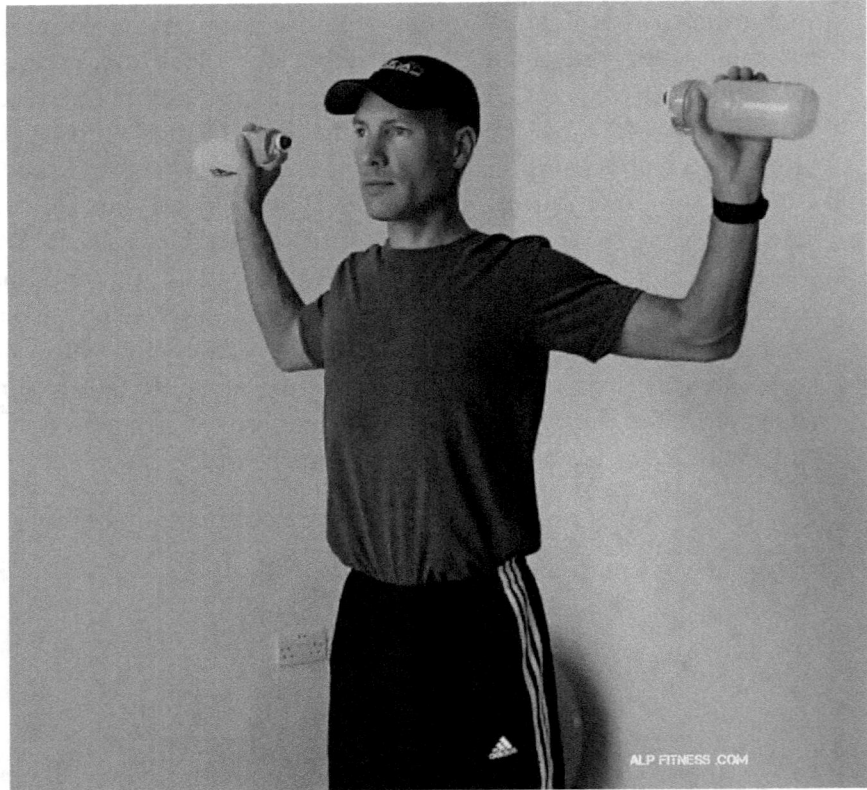

Figure 6-19. Abducted external rotation (ending point)

Behind the Neck Cord Pull-Apart

This exercise targets the lower trapezius, which plays an important role in stabilizing your shoulder blades through upward scapular rotation. The motion is similar to that of a lat pulldown. Grab a stretch cord in both hands and raise them directly over your head; remove any slack from the cord so that you start with some tension. From this starting position, lower your arms by leading with your elbows. As you lower your arms, bringing the cord behind your neck, it will feel like you are pulling the cord apart as you squeeze the shoulder blades together. At the end of the pull, hold it for 2 seconds; then return to the starting position and repeat.

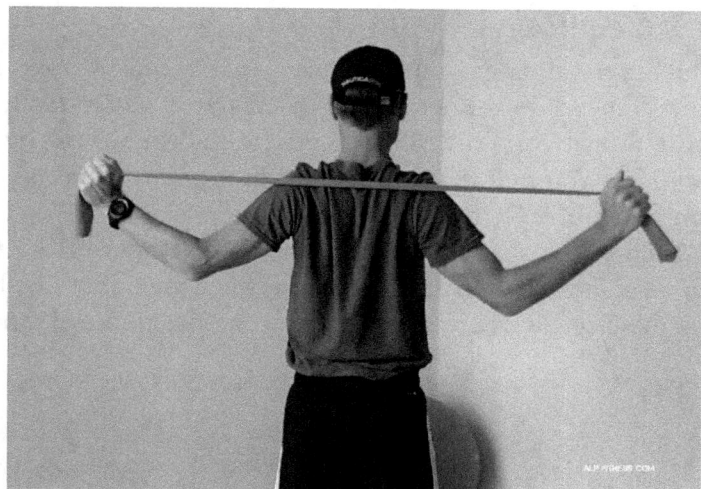

Figure 6-20. Behind the neck cord pull-apart

Hitchhiker

This exercise targets the muscles that stabilize your shoulders and your shoulder blades. Lie on the ground face down. Place your arms out to the side with thumbs up; this is your starting position. From here, squeeze together your shoulder blades as you lift your thumbs toward the ceiling. Slowly return and repeat.

Variation. A variation of the lying hitchhiker is to stand on one leg and bend forward with the other leg behind you to put yourself in a horizontal position. From this position, perform the exercise as described above.

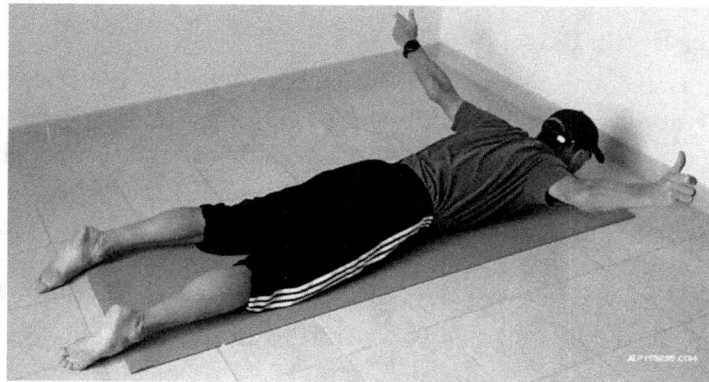

Figure 6-21. Hitchhiker

Stretch Cord Row

This exercise targets the muscles that stabilize your shoulder blades. You can do this sitting on an exercise ball or standing. Lean forward to get into the starting position. From there, keep your elbows in as you pull the stretch cord to a point between your belly button and rib cage; this is the finishing position. As you pull the cord, keep your palms up and squeeze the shoulder blades together. As you end, imagine pinching a coin between your shoulder blades to hold it in place. Slowly return to the starting position and repeat.

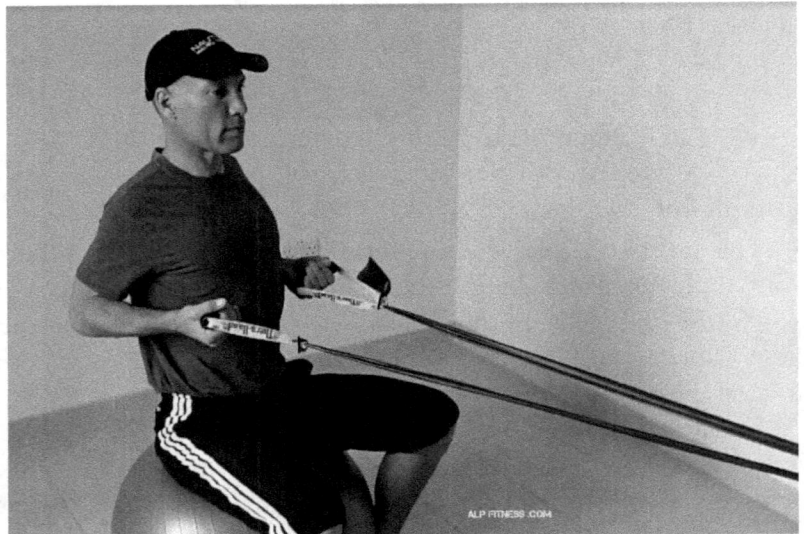

Figure 6-22. Stretch Cord Row

Water Bottle Raise

This exercise targets the infraspinatus, which is used in abduction. As with all exercises described here, start by putting your shoulder blades in your back pockets and keep them there throughout the exercise. Stand straight with arms to your side. Raise your arms up to the side so they are shoulder level, turn the thumbs up, and move your arms forward 1-2 feet. This is the up position. Now slowly lower the arms and repeat the raising and lowering from this position. Keep the thumbs up the whole time as if you are holding a glass of water.

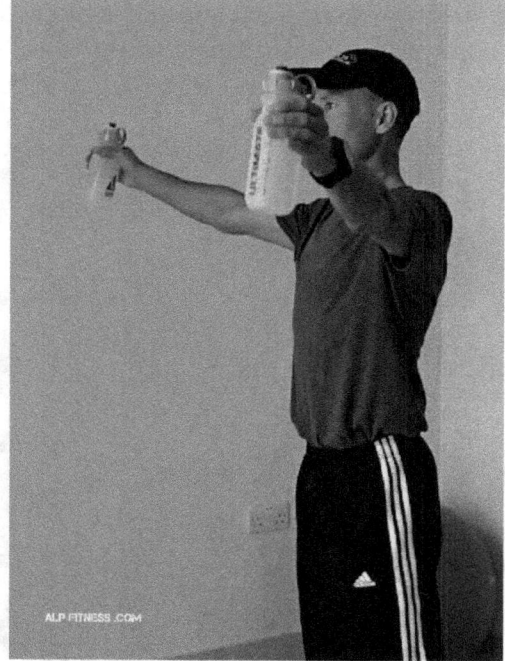

Figure 6-23. Water Bottle Raise

Pushup "Plus" Rounded Finish

In addition to targeting your chest muscles like a regular pushup, this exercise also targets the serratus anterior, which holds the shoulder blades to the rib cage (to prevent what is termed "scapular winging"). In this exercise, you perform a regular pushup but when you get to the end you keep going. As you continue pushing past the normal end point, your shoulders will round forward a bit as you raise your back. Hold for 2 seconds; then return to the down position and repeat. To get a feel for this exercise, start by performing the pushup against a wall. Then progress to a pushup from the knees. When ready, you can do the pushup from the regular position.

Ball on wall

This exercise targets the muscles that stabilize your shoulder blades along with your internal and external rotators. Stand arm's length away from a wall. Squeeze your shoulder blades and put them in your back pocket (yes, you should know the drill by now!). Take a tennis or lacrosse ball and push it against the wall so the palm of your hand pins it to the wall. Make a small clockwise circle for 15 seconds;

then reverse direction for 15 seconds. Continue this for up to 2 minutes or until you can no longer keep your shoulder blades together or hold the ball up. Repeat with the other arm.

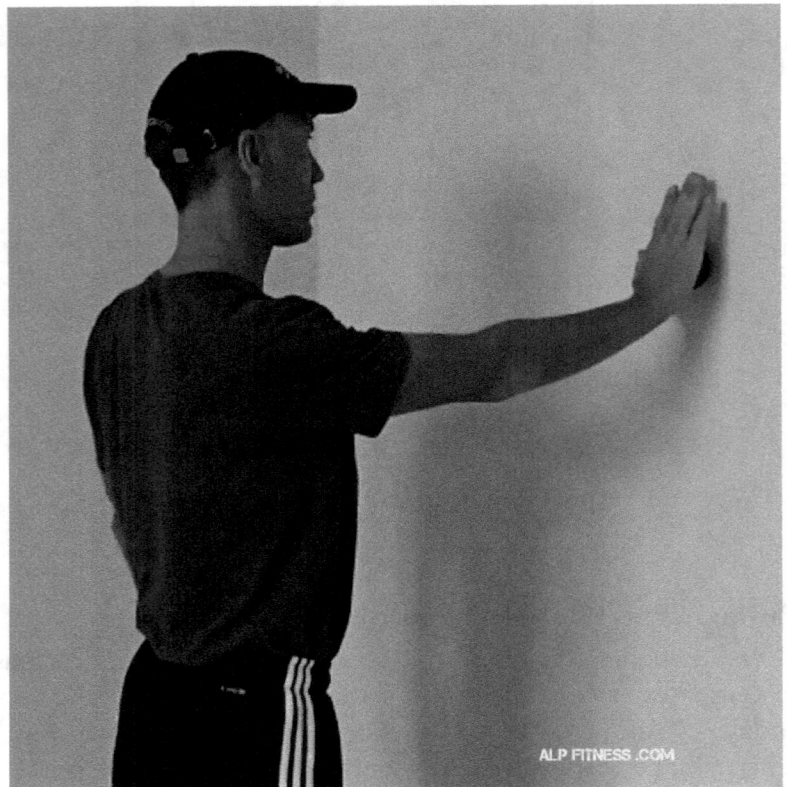

Figure 6-24. Ball on Wall

Chest Stretch

This stretch targets your chest. Standing with your face against a wall, put one arm out to the side so it is parallel to the ground. Now bend the elbow up 10-15°. Use your opposite hand to push the other side of your body off the wall. You should feel a stretch in your chest. Hold for 30 seconds to 3 minutes; then repeat on the other side. You can also do this stretch lying on the floor in a prone position.

Complete Workouts

Strength (Core/Legs – Full Version)

Perform one set of each exercise, moving from one to the next in a circuit. As you advance, repeat the circuit 2-3 times. Add weight/resistance or reps as needed to perform each exercise to fatigue. Always perform exercises with perfect form.

1. Good mornings – 8-12 reps
2. Squats* – 8-12 reps
3. Superman – 8-12 reps
4. Glute bridge* – 8-12 reps
5. Front plank – 30-90 seconds
6. Donkey kicks – 8-12 per leg
7. Side plank – 30 seconds per side
8. Hip abductions (lying) – 8-12 reps per leg

*As you advance, perform single leg squats and single leg glute bridges.

Strength (Core/Legs – Introductory Short Version #1)

Take 10 minutes out of the day when you have a break to do these exercises. Perform the exercises in a circuit, moving from one to the next:

1. Squat (Hip Hinge) - 30-60 seconds
2. Front Plank - 30-60 seconds
3. Donkey Kicks - 30 seconds per leg
4. Side Plank - 30 seconds per side
5. Hip Abductions (Lying) - 30 seconds per leg

Complete the circuit 2 times for a 10 minute workout. You can increase the number of times through the circuit (or the time spent on each exercise) to lengthen the workout.

Strength (Core/Legs – Introductory Short Version #2)

Take 10 minutes out of the day when you have a break to do these exercises. Perform the exercises in a circuit, moving from one to the next:

1. Good Mornings - 20 seconds (or 8-15 reps)
2. Standing Leg Abduction - 20 seconds each leg (or 8-15 reps)
3. Front Plank - 30-60 seconds
4. Donkey Kicks - 20 seconds each leg (or 8-15 reps)
5. Glute Bridge - 20 seconds (or 8-15 reps)

Complete the circuit 3-4 times for a 10 minute workout. You can increase the number of times through the circuit (or the time spent on each exercise) to lengthen the workout.

Strength (Core/Legs – Advanced Short Version #1)

Take 10 minutes out of the day when you have a break to do these exercises. Perform the exercises in a circuit, moving from one to the next:

1. Good Mornings - 20 seconds (or 8-15 reps)
2. Squat - 20 seconds (or 8-15 reps)
3. Front Plank with Leg Extension – 30-60 seconds in plank while doing 1-2 x 8-12 reps of leg extension each leg
4. Side Plank with Hip Abductions – 30 seconds per side while doing 8-12 reps of hip abductions

Complete the circuit 3 times for a 10 minute workout. You can increase the number of times through the circuit (or the time spent on each exercise) to lengthen the workout.

Strength (Core/Legs – Advanced Short Version #2)

Take 10 minutes out of the day when you have a break to do these exercises. Perform the exercises in a circuit, moving from one to the next:

1. Superman – 20-30 seconds (or 8-20 reps)
2. Front Plank – 30-60 seconds
3. Back Extension – 30 seconds (or 8-15 reps)
4. Front Plank with Straight Leg Extension – 30-60 seconds in plank while doing 1-2 x 8-12 reps of leg extension each leg
5. Glute Bridge (Single Leg) – 20 seconds (or 8-12 reps) per leg

Complete the circuit 2-3 times for a 10 minute workout. You can increase the number of times through the circuit (or the time spent on each exercise) to lengthen the workout.

Strength (Core/Legs – Advanced 30-minute Workout)

Warm up for 3-5 min with some dynamic walking and/or skips:

1. High Knee Walk
2. Hurdle Walk
3. Straight Leg Walk
4. Loosening Skips

Perform the exercises in circuits, moving from one to the next, as outlined below.

Circuit #1 – Perform circuit 3 times
1. Good Mornings - 20 seconds (or 8-15 reps)
2. Squat - 20 seconds (or 8-15 reps)

Take 15-30 seconds rest

Circuit #2 – Perform circuit 3 times
1. Donkey Kicks - 20 seconds each leg (or 8-12 reps)
2. Hip Abductions (Lying) - 20 seconds each side (or 8-12 reps)

Take 15-30 seconds rest

Circuit #3 – Perform circuit 3 times
1. Superman – 20 seconds (or 8-12 reps)
2. Back Extension – 20 seconds (or 8-12 reps)

Take 15-30 seconds rest

Circuit #4 – Perform circuit 3 times
1. Front Plank - 30-60 seconds
2. Side Plank - 30 seconds each side

Take 15-30 seconds rest

Circuit #5 – Perform circuit 3 times
1. Front Plank with Straight Leg Extension – 30-60 seconds in plank while doing 1-2 x 8-12 reps of leg extension each leg
2. Side Plank with Hip Abductions (Lying) – 30 seconds per side of side plank while doing 8-12 reps of hip abductions
3. Glute Bridge (Single Leg) – 20 seconds (or 8-12 reps) per leg

Take 15-30 seconds rest

Finish with single leg balance drills. Do 20 seconds per leg, alternating back and forth 3 times.

Strength (Shoulders/Back – Full Workout)

Perform one set of each exercise, moving from one to the next in a circuit. As you advance, repeat the circuit 2-3 times. Add weight/resistance or reps as needed to perform each exercise to fatigue. Always perform exercises with perfect form.

1. Behind neck cord pull apart – 8-12 reps
2. External rotation – 8-12 reps
3. Hitchhiker – 8-12 reps
4. Stretch cord row – 8-12 reps
5. Water bottle raise – 8-12 reps
6. Pushup "plus" rounded finish – 8-12 reps
7. Ball on wall – 1-2 min per shoulder
8. Chest stretch – 30 seconds per side

For exercises that have variations, choose one of the variations. For exercises that have progressions (e.g. pushup "plus"), begin with the initial progression and advance when you are ready.

7
RECOVERY AND NUTRITION

As stated in the introduction, it is easy to overlook recovery. Yet, as evident from the earlier discussion of the stress-response-adaptation process that underlies fitness gains, recovery is central to that process. After all, your gains are made during recovery between training sessions, not during the training sessions. Without adequate recovery, you can't make those fitness gains. This chapter provides tips on how to monitor and make the most of your recovery. In addition, it provides general tips that every athlete should know about nutrition both during and outside of training and racing.

Stress is Stress

Remember that training stress is not the only type of stress you encounter as an athlete. In addition to the demands of physical training required to produce overload, there are various levels of stress associated with work, school, and other aspects of one's life. If you are faced with a looming deadline at work that has placed some pressure on your shoulders, the extra stress in that area of your life can impact the amount of training stress you are able to handle until the work deadline has passed. The key take away message here is to not get frustrated if you find yourself unable to train at the level you're accustomed to when you are under greater loads of stress in other areas of your life. It is important to recognize this basic point and to adjust your training accordingly. Again, *it is not the absolute training load that matters, but the training load that your body can handle that matters.*

Easy Means Easy

Another important mantra to keep in mind is to *keep the hard days hard and the easy days easy*. Remember, training effects are achieved by applying an appropriate stimulus and then backing off so the body can positively adapt. Days on which harder workouts are scheduled are important for applying that stimulus. Key workouts are therefore an essential part of your training, and you want to be able to go into them capable of hitting the targeted training at the prescribed intensity level. And the best way to ensure you are ready to work hard and get the most out of those key workouts is to pay attention to your recovery on the easy days. In other words, you often need to *go easy to become fast*.

It can sometimes be tempting to push the pace a bit on those recovery days when you are feeling good. "Why not?" you might think to yourself, "If I gain fitness through hard training; then I should train hard all the time." What usually happens, though, is that those easy workouts that morph into not-quite-easy workouts end up taking you into a dead-end zone where you are neither going fast enough to achieve a proper overload nor slow enough to adequately recover. Such a situation might be described as a wasted workout or junk miles. At best, you might carry a little extra fatigue into your next hard day. At worst, you might be unable to hit the training target on the next hard day due to inadequate recovery going into it. Instead of achieving the desired training effect to ratchet up your fitness level, you then need to wait until you are better recovered before trying again. The take away point is to use your recovery workouts for just that—recovery. They are just as essential to your training as your hard days.

Tuning into Heart Rate

Heart rate can provide an important window into your state of recovery, providing signs on when to continue with planned training or when to readjust the workout.

One sign that you may need further recovery workouts instead of that planned higher intensity one is how your heart rate responds during a training session. Let's say you are pushing the envelope with hard training and enter into a workout knowing you're close to the edge of overreaching. After you do your initial warmup you dive into a set of intervals at a higher intensity level. Although a bit sluggish at first, you seem to be close to the target according to your pace. However, you are unable to elevate your heart rate into the target zone, a fact confirmed by your heart rate monitor. In this case, an inability to elevate your heart rate when you've clearly upped the intensity indicates your body has not recovered from previous sessions. Heed the sign and turn that interval session into a short recovery workout. Then go home and conscientiously facilitate further recovery over the next few days before returning to higher intensity training.

Ideally, though, you would like a way to determine how recovered you are before even starting a workout. This is where morning heart rate readings can prove instructive. A simple approach is to take your heart rate each morning before getting out of bed. Keep track of the average over time. If your heart rate is 5-10 beats higher than average on a given morning, this is a sign you may need more rest and recovery that day. It could also mean your body is fighting a virus, in which case eliminating stress in the form of hard training can give your body a chance to nip in the bud any sort of oncoming illness.

Another variation of the resting heart rate test is to take your orthostatic heart rate. You can do this in the morning upon waking or after lying down and resting for at least 15 minutes. Start by taking your resting heart rate while lying down. Next, stand up and take your heart rate. Subtract the difference between the lying and standing readings. If the difference is more than 15-20 beats; then additional recovery is called for.

These simple techniques can provide measurable insight into your state of recovery. The more experience you gain in using these techniques, the better you will be able to read the nuanced signs of overtraining.

Supplemental Work

In outlining the ABCs of training in chapter 1, I mentioned the importance of *consistent supplemental work*. In addition to form drills and functional strength exercises, supplemental work also includes preventive care to enhance flexibility and mobility. Together, functional strength work along with preventive care effectively provides you with a "prehab" program to keep your body healthy. Doing prehab can help you avoid the dreaded "rehab" program of an injured athlete.

A vital element of prehab involves keeping your connective tissues healthy. Connective tissues are found everywhere, including the tendons that connect muscles to bones, the fasciae that surround muscle groups, and the endomysium that surrounds individual muscle cells. Connective tissues are comprised of a protein called collagen. When collagen fibers run parallel, like straws in a box, everything works the way it should. Muscles can contract without obstructions and tissues are able to withstand the stress loads placed upon them through physical activity. But the simple fact is that training breaks down the body. If it didn't, there would be no opportunity to grow stronger through positive adaptations during the rebuilding phase.

As long as the tissues heal properly, then mobility is maintained and the body can continue to function at a high level of performance. But complete tissue rebuilding can take up to a few weeks while training takes place on an ongoing basis. That means there are ample opportunities for tissues to rebuild in a less than effective manner. Instead of the collagen fibers lining up in parallel like straws in a box, the fibers begin to look more like a pile of straws arranged in a haphazard fashion. This is when adhesions, scars or trigger points begin to develop.

One of the easiest and most effective means to ensure the healthy rebuilding of the body in between workouts is to use self-massage techniques. All you need is a few minutes each day along with some useful tools that include a foam roller, rolling massage stick, lacrosse ball, and golf ball. A daily once over of the major areas of the body allows you to prevent or to at least notice trigger points when they first begin to develop so you can eliminate them before they get worse.

Recovery Tools

Given the importance of recovery, it is wise to pay conscientious attention to recovery in between workouts to enhance the process and prepare for your next training session. Fortunately, there are several tools that athletes have at their disposal to aid recovery. Many of these tools involve aiding blood circulation to clear muscles of inflammation and metabolic waste that contributes to soreness and fatigue.

A popular and traditional method to aid recovery is a light sports massage. There's a reason Tour de France cyclists head for the massage table after racing each day. Massage aids recovery by increasing circulation, increases joint flexibility, and relieves tension in overused muscles. Deep tissue work has its place in the recovery cycle, but nothing beats a light flush of the muscles so that you can get back to it with fresher legs the next day.

Although few athletes have access to a massage therapist on a daily basis, anyone can easily integrate self-massage into their daily routines. With the advent of foam rollers (cylinders made of dense foam, 5 to 6 inches in diameter and a foot or more in length), athletes now have access to an essential tool for performing self-massage (a.k.a. "poor man's massage"). Similar to the work done by a massage therapist to break up adhesions in the muscle tissue, an athlete can apply varying amounts of body weight to the foam roller to work out the trigger points. In addition to foam rollers, rolling massage sticks, lacrosse balls, and golf balls can all be used to pinpoint trouble spots. Keep these tools next to the desk during the workday, and use them during breaks to work out the tensions from sitting. Even 10 minutes a day can be beneficial.

Another recovery aid is the cold water plunge. By increasing circulation, cold plunges can speed the removal of toxins associated with muscle damage. Even a plunge of only 30 to 45 seconds can have a benefit. If you don't have access to a cold mountain stream or an ice bath; then set the faucet to 'cold' for the last few minutes of your shower. Especially during the warm summer months, there's nothing more refreshing than a cold shower after a tough workout.

Continuing with the theme of "all things that aid blood circulation help recovery," add compression sleeves to that list. It is no mystery why the medical field had long been using compression garments with surgery patients before athletes discovered them. Wearing compression socks/sleeves can improve venous return from those hammered calves. While the jury is still out on whether wearing them during training/racing can help performance, they certainly do have positive benefits for aiding recovery between workouts.

Of the many tools available to help athletes recover, active compression—and not just passive compression as with the compression sleeves—is one of the most effective. It has also been used in the medical field for years and is now becoming the latest weapon in the arsenal of elite endurance athletes. Devices such as the Recovery Pump or NormaTec system consist of a small box (the pump) that plugs into a typical wall electrical outlet, and two "boots" that connect to the pump via small-diameter hoses. The boots cover the leg from the toes to the top of the thigh. Once you slip on the boots and zip them up, the medical grade device inflates sequentially from the toes to the base of the buttocks. The pumping action mimics the natural muscle pumps in the legs during exercise. Both the Recovery Pump and NormaTec systems can be pricey, but they are effective and worth the investment for serious athletes.

Active Recovery

Recovery is not always a passive endeavor even if one often thinks of it that way. Your recovery begins the minute you have completed the last work interval during your hard training session. High intensity activity leads to the accumulation of lactic acid in the bloodstream, which can lead to that heavy muscle feeling. The easiest way to begin clearing away blood lactate is to swim, bike or run at a moderate aerobic pace (i.e. Zone 2) at the end of your workout. Low level aerobic activity turns that lactate into energy and removes it from the muscles.

Although sometimes a day spent lying on the couch and napping is just what the body needs, on many "rest days" the body will benefit from some type of activity. Walks, yoga or other light activity that gets the body moving stimulates the lymph and circulatory systems, which are important to the recovery process. The key is to keep the activity easy. If you choose to get in the water, on the bike, or go for a run on a "rest day," then limit that session to a short, easy warm up—just enough to raise the body temperature, produce a bit of sweat and get the blood flowing.

Remember, fitness gains occur during recovery. A proper recovery allows your body a chance to adapt from a hard training session, and will ensure that it is ready to get the most out of the next one.

Sleep

The recommended amount of sleep for healthy adults is 7 to 9 hours per day. According to a 2012 study by the Centers for Disease Control (CDC), 30 percent of American adults are "sleep deprived," meaning they sleep less than 6 hours each day—leaving them vulnerable to adverse health and safety effects.

As any athlete in training knows, skipping on sleep is not conducive to optimal athletic performance. Train as much as you want, but without adequate sleep the body is unable to absorb the training. As you know by now, that is because physiological adaptations occur during the recovery periods in between training bouts. Without rest and recovery, the body continues to break down rather than to rebuild.

Athletes in training should aim for the recommended 7 to 9 hours of sleep each day plus additional hours depending upon their activity level. Here are a few rules of thumb for determining how much extra sleep to include in your weekly schedule.

Rule of Thumb #1. A good general rule of thumb is to take the number of hours you train each week, move the decimal point one place to the left, and add that amount of time to your daily sleep. For example, if you train 10 hours a week; then aim for an extra hour of sleep each day. If you normally find yourself needing 8 hours of sleep; then you would bump that up to 9 hours.

Rule of Thumb #2. This rule of thumb is more specific to running. Here, take the number of miles you run per week and aim for the same number of extra minutes of sleep per night. For example, if you run 30 miles per week in your training; then aim for an extra 30 minutes per day of sleep. If you normally find yourself needing 7.5 hours of sleep per night; then you would bump that up to 8 hours.

To be sure, these are simply rules of thumb, and you will need to pinpoint your own particular needs based on individual circumstances. But they do help to underscore the key take away point that *you need more sleep during heavy training periods.*

At the minimum, make sure you get the recommended baseline of 7 to 9 hours per day; then add in extra time according to your activity level and individual needs. If you're training 20 hours a week; then sleeping 10 hours a day is not a luxury—it's a necessity.

Keep in mind, extra sleep need not occur only at night. Naps during the day, particularly after intense workouts, are another good way to ensure you get the rest you need. At the very least, dedicate that extra time to rest and relaxation even if it's not a full sleep. Your body will thank you and you will put yourself in a position to feel better both on and off the race course.

Nutrition and Hydration during Exercise

Just like when driving a car, the amount of fuel you burn during exercise depends upon how fast you are going—that is, your intensity level. At lower intensity levels, your body burns more fat as an energy source. As the intensity rises, more carbohydrates are burned. Note that the body always draws on both sources of fuel; it is just the relative amounts that shift with intensity.

As the saying goes, fat burns in carbohydrate's flame. This means your body requires a certain amount of carbohydrates to maintain aerobic oxidation. The body can draw upon the carbohydrates stored in your muscles and liver, which is called "glycogen." The body can also draw upon carbohydrates you eat while exercising. In both cases, carbohydrates are converted to glucose in the bloodstream, which is the form your exercising muscles utilize to provide you with energy.

How much glycogen does your body store? Although it will vary depending upon recent workouts, eating patterns and your personal fitness level, a body typically stores enough glycogen to provide energy for up to a few hours of moderate activity. Obviously, the more "metabolically efficient" you are—meaning your body utilizes more fat while sparing glycogen—the longer you can go without needing to ingest any additional carbohydrates to keep the flame burning. This is the logic behind the recent emphasis among endurance athletes—especially ultra-runners and long course triathletes—on becoming more metabolically efficient.

One step to improve your metabolic efficiency is to forgo nutritional supplements on most of your long workout sessions during early base training. Since we are accustomed to having a steady supply of sugary foods in our modern diet, this can be a shock for some. Abstain from eating for at least the first 90 minutes of your workout. Try to extend that past 90 minutes and eventually up to 2 hours or more. Experiment for yourself and notice what your typical end point is before you feel you must eat.

As you move closer to racing season or begin to up the intensity of some of those longer workout sessions, then experiment with the type of nutritional products you plan to use while racing. Sport drinks and gels tend to work better for higher intensity, shorter races because they absorb faster. For longer events, energy bars or solid food can be an option depending upon your personal preference. Be sure to practice during your training with the type of products that will be available on the race course so there are no surprises.

How much should you ingest while racing? Typically, most bodies are able to digest about 200-300 calories per hour during racing. That's the equivalent of two to three gels or a single energy bar—less if you are washing it down with a sport drink. Experiment during training to pinpoint your own needs and tolerance levels.

Keep in mind that for races that you can finish within 75 minutes, you shouldn't need to worry about energy replacement. Simply drink water as needed and focus on racing. Save the eating for the post-race refreshments. Many can even race at a decent intensity level for up to 2 hours without needing to worry about energy replacement.

But for longer races, aim to start titrating your fuel intake about a half hour to an hour into the race. It is best to titrate this evenly throughout the race to maintain a consistent blood sugar level. This means setting up a feeding schedule—for example, every 15 minutes or every 20 minutes or every 30 minutes—to follow throughout your race. Keep in mind that eating more than your body can handle is just as deleterious to performance as not eating enough. Know your needs and refuel accordingly.

You might find it helpful to set an alarm on your watch to beep every 20 minutes to remind you to eat/drink on cue. This is particularly helpful for long course events where you spend the better part of a day out on the course. The key to success in those types of events—such as an Ironman triathlon—is to stave off the energy depletion that necessarily occurs over the course of the day as your body simply burns more calories than you are able to replace. This is okay up to a point, remember, because much of that energy will come from your stored fat and glycogen reserves; but you will need to replace some carbohydrates along the way to keep the flame burning to utilize your ample stores of fat (even lean athletes have ample fat storage to get through a long day of activity).

For long events and races in warmer weather, hydration and electrolyte replacement becomes necessary. Simply drinking water alone is insufficient because it lacks the sodium (and other minerals) lost in sweat. Drinking too much water without taking in sodium can result in the deadly condition of hyponatremia (literally, "low sodium"). Sport drinks that provide a balanced amount of electrolytes are a good choice for replacing both fluids and electrolytes. Salt or electrolyte tablets in conjunction with drinking water are another option.

If you use a sport drink, be mindful of how much (and what type of) sugar it contains. Not all sport drinks are created equal. This is where you need to experiment with products before race day to determine what works best for you. Sometimes the sport drink provided at aid stations is mixed at either higher or lower concentration levels than what you buy off the shelf in the store. If it's overly concentrated, you may need to drink extra water to dilute it. Race day can throw many surprises your way, but if you know your needs given the type of conditions you encounter then you will be able to adapt accordingly.

As a general rule of thumb, drink to thirst. For any race, you will lose some body weight from sweating; and this need not be completely replaced during the race itself. Certainly, sweat loss is less a problem during shorter events; and severe dehydration must be avoided. During longer events, setting up a drinking schedule—such as every 15 minutes or 20 minutes—will allow you to titrate your fluid and electrolyte replacement for maximum effectiveness. Different weather conditions obviously dictate the amount of fluids and electrolytes you need to replace, so adjust accordingly.

Nutrition and Hydration after Exercise

In exercise bouts that last over an hour, muscle glycogen (the body's carbohydrate stores) become depleted and needs to be replaced. It is best to start this process within a half hour (or at least within an hour) after exercise by consuming around a half gram of carbohydrate per pound of body weight. For example, a 160 pound triathlete would target about 80 grams of carbohydrate, which translates into a snack of 320 calories (for example, a banana with almond butter). Your choice of snack will depend upon your personal preferences, but keep the snack healthy and you will start your recovery on the right track. Even better, schedule one of your main meals after a big workout.

One of the body's reactions to intense exercise is inflammation. Reducing inflammation is therefore an important part of the recovery process. Essential fatty acids help to decrease the body's inflammation response, and should be an important part of your daily diet. In particular, the omega-3 fatty acid is often underrepresented in typical diets. Cold water fish (e.g. tuna, salmon) and flax seeds/oil are excellent sources of omega-3. Yet another food item that has anti-inflammatory properties is pineapple—specifically, the enzyme bromelain that is found in pineapple. Instead of reaching for a soda, try a glass of cold pineapple juice instead. It also provides a nice dose of carbohydrates to help replenish depleted glycogen stores in the muscles.

Nutrition to Support Fitness and Health

Just as sleep is a vital component of supporting fitness and health, so is a healthy diet. When it comes to eating well, you can navigate today's world of highly processed food loaded with added sugar by keeping in mind that the best sources of nutrition are whole foods with minimal processing (rather than pre-packaged meals and snack items). Eating a wide variety of whole foods ensures you are getting the nutrients you need to stay fueled and healthy. In addition, drink enough water throughout the day so that your urine is the color of straw.

At meals, aim for a mix of lean protein and healthy fat with your carbohydrates. Whole foods are always better than processed foods. Instead of white bread or white rice, opt for whole grain bread or long grain wild rice. Avoid foods with added sugars; nature provides plenty of simple carbs in the form of whole fruits and vegetables (fresh or frozen). Aim for a colorful plate with leafy greens and other veggies. And keep in mind that there's nothing wrong with healthy fat. In fact, healthy sources of fat are a vital part of your nutritional needs—think avocados, olive oil, salmon, flax seeds, almonds, walnuts. Good fat—along with fiber—helps to sate your hunger so you can actually stop eating sooner (and even consume fewer calories) than if you're looking only to carbohydrates (especially simple ones) to achieve satiety. Finally, remember to slow down and chew your food thoroughly. Enjoy the process of both preparing and consuming the food that drives your health and performance.

PART IV

TRAINING PLANS & WORKOUT LIBRARY

8
TRAINING PLANS

The training plans in this chapter are arranged into 4-week training blocks. Each training block corresponds to a different phase of the base-build-peak progression (the first two blocks are dedicated to base training):

1 – Establish Your Base
2 – Develop Your Base
3 – Build Upon Your Base
4 – Peak for Your Race

Depending upon the overall length of your season, you can repeat training blocks as needed before advancing to the next phase of your training. So, think of these as building blocks that you can use to build your own custom training plan.

Although distances/durations are provided for each workout, adjust up/down according to your personal starting point and rate of progression. Start by noting the first week's training hours. Does it match the typical training volume you have used in the past? If not, adjust the weekly training hours up/down to match your starting point. Based on changes you make to the first week's training hours, adjust the rest of the plan's weekly hours.

You can use these building blocks as a blueprint to train for triathlons of various distances. Modify the duration of your long run and long bike—along with your overall training volume—according to your race goals and experience level.

Each 4-week training block uses a 3-up/1-down periodization schedule. But you can modify these to a 2-up/1-down schedule. For all but the peak training block, simply delete the third week. The peak training block provides a 3-week taper to a target race, followed by a post-race recovery week. Each training block provides specific guidelines on how to use it and where to go next once you've completed it.

The plans are balanced with an equal number of workouts per discipline each week. The training blocks in the first section consist of two discipline-specific workouts per week—that is, two swims, two bikes, two runs. Those in the next section consist of three discipline-specific workouts per week. Those in the final section consist of four discipline-specific workouts per week. You can always add/subtract workouts, but start with a plan that most closely matches how many discipline-specific workouts you typically do each week. Keep in mind that the plans with more discipline-specific workouts allow for an overall greater training volume.

Depending on your strengths and weaknesses, you may want to tweak the number of workouts per discipline or the ratio of training hours assigned to each discipline. For example, if you come from a running background but are new to swimming, you might choose to increase the frequency of your swims since frequency builds skill. You can then either leave the overall swim training volume the same—in which case you simply redistribute that volume across the additional swims—or you can simply dedicate additional time to swimming each week, perhaps in place of time spent training your strongest discipline.

For detailed workout descriptions, see the library of swim, bike and run workouts in the three chapters that follow.

If you use TrainingPeaks to schedule, track and monitor your training, you can purchase these plans—complete with detailed workout descriptions and tips for modifying the interval workouts — from the TrainingPeaks store to load directly into your calendar. See the Alp Fitness website for links (alpfitness.com/training-plans/).

2 Workouts/Discipline/Week

1 – Establish Your Base

Welcome to your first phase of base training. This 4-week training block provides you with a 3-up/1-down periodization schedule. You can change it to a 2-up/1-down schedule by simply deleting the third week.

The last week of the training block is a recovery week with testing scheduled at the end. The tests allow you to monitor your progress and (if needed) recalibrate your training zones.

Suggested distances/durations for each workout are provided; but you should adjust up or down according to your personal starting point.

Rearrange the workouts on your calendar as needed. Do so with an eye toward maintaining a consistent spacing between workouts of a particular discipline and balancing harder days with easier days.

This training block can be repeated multiple times early in the base training part of your season as you increase your training volume. As a rule of thumb, add about 10 percent to your training volume each time you repeat the training block.

Week 1 – Establish Your Base (2 Workouts/Discipline)

Day	Workout		Duration
Monday	Rest day		
Tuesday	Swim (Easy with drills)		0:30
	Strength (Shoulders/back)		0:20
Wednesday	Bike (Easy with drills)		0:30
Thursday	Run (Easy with drills)		0:30
	Strength (Core/legs)		0:20
Friday	Swim (Aerobic base 100s)		0:30
Saturday	Bike (Endurance with short sprints)		1:00
Sunday	Run (Endurance with striders)		0:45
	or Run (Endurance with short hills)		
Summary	Total	4:25	
	Swim	1:00	
	Bike	1:30	
	Run	1:15	

Strength   0:40

Week 2 – Establish Your Base (2 Workouts/Discipline)

Monday	Rest day	
Tuesday	Swim (Easy with drills)	0:30
	Strength (Shoulders/back)	0:20
Wednesday	Bike (Easy with drills)	0:30
Thursday	Run (Easy with drills)	0:30
	Strength (Core/legs)	0:20
Friday	Swim (Aerobic base 200s)	0:45
Saturday	Bike (Endurance with short sprints)	1:20
Sunday	Run (Endurance with striders)	0:55
	or Run (Endurance with short hills)	
Summary	Total 5:10	
	Swim 1:15	
	Bike 1:50	
	Run 1:25	
	Strength 0:40	

Week 3 – Establish Your Base (2 Workouts/Discipline)

Monday	Rest day	
Tuesday	Swim (Easy with drills)	0:30
	Strength (Shoulders/back)	0:20
Wednesday	Bike (Easy with drills)	0:30
Thursday	Run (Easy with drills)	0:30
	Strength (Core/legs)	0:20

Friday	Swim (Aerobic base 500s)	1:00
Saturday	Bike (Endurance with short sprints)	1:45
Sunday	Run (Endurance with striders) or Run (Endurance with short hills)	1:05
Summary	Total 5:10 Swim 1:15 Bike 1:50 Run 1:25 Strength 0:40	

Week 4 – Recovery and Testing

Monday	Rest day	
Tuesday	Swim (Easy with drills)	0:20
Wednesday	Bike (Easy with drills)	0:20
Thursday	Run (Easy with drills)	0:20
Friday	Rest day	
Saturday	Run (20-min LT time trial)	0:45
Sunday	Swim (1,000-yd/m time trial)	0:45
Summary	Total 2:30 Swim 1:05 Bike 0:20 Run 1:05	

The Next Step

Depending upon the overall shape of your season, you can either repeat this training block or advance to the next training block of the 4-step series.

If you repeat this training block, increase your training volume by approximately 10 percent. When you advance to the next block, adjust your first week's training volume so it is no more than 10 percent above where you finished the third week of this one.

2 – Develop Your Base

Welcome to your second phase of base training. This 4-week training block provides you with a 3-up/1-down periodization schedule. You can change it to a 2-up/1-down schedule by simply deleting the third week.

The last week of the training block is a recovery week with testing scheduled at the end. The tests allow you to monitor your progress and (if needed) recalibrate your training zones.

Suggested distances/durations for each workout are provided; but you should adjust the first week's training volume so it is no more than 10 percent above the third week's volume of the previous training block. From there, either maintain or slightly increase the volume of weeks two and three.

Rearrange the workouts on your calendar as needed. Do so with an eye toward maintaining a consistent spacing between workouts of a particular discipline and balancing harder days with easier days.

This training block can be repeated multiple times during the late base training part of your season as you increase your training volume and/or time spent at threshold pace.

Week 1 – Develop Your Base (2 Workouts/Discipline)

Day	Workout	Duration
Monday	Rest day	
Tuesday	Swim (Fartlek 25s, drills)	0:40
	Strength (Shoulders/back)	0:20
Wednesday	Bike (Easy with short sprints)	0:50
Thursday	Run (Easy with striders, drills)	0:40
	Strength (Core/legs)	0:20

Friday	Swim (Base tempo 100s)	1:00
Saturday	Bike (Sub-LT 20-in tempo)	1:40
Sunday	Run (Sub-LT cruise intervals 8/2)	1:00

Summary	Total	6:30
	Swim	1:40
	Bike	2:30
	Run	1:40
	Strength	0:40

Week 2 – Develop Your Base (2 Workouts/Discipline)

Monday	Rest day	
Tuesday	Swim (Fartlek 25s, drills)	0:40
	Strength (Shoulders/back)	0:20
Wednesday	Bike (Easy with short sprints)	0:50
Thursday	Run (Easy with striders, drills)	0:40
	Strength (Core/legs)	0:20
Friday	Swim (LT Cruise 300s)	1:00
Saturday	Bike (Sub-LT cruise intervals 8/2)	1:50
Sunday	Run (Sub-LT 20-in tempo)	1:10

Summary	Total	6:50
	Swim	1:40
	Bike	2:40
	Run	1:50
	Strength	0:40

Week 3 – Develop Your Base (2 Workouts/Discipline)

| Monday | Rest day |

Tuesday	Swim (Fartlek 25s, drills)	0:40
	Strength (Shoulders/back)	0:20
Wednesday	Bike (Easy with short sprints)	0:50
Thursday	Run (Easy with striders, drills)	0:40
	Strength (Core/legs)	0:20
Friday	Swim (LT Cruise 500s)	1:00
Saturday	Bike (Sub-LT 20-min tempo) or Bike (Cruise intervals)	2:00
Sunday	Run (Sub-LT cruise intervals 8/2) or Run (Sub-LT 20-min tempo)	1:20
Summary	Total 7:10	
	Swim 1:40	
	Bike 2:50	
	Run 2:00	
	Strength 0:40	

Week 4 – Recovery and Testing

Monday	Rest day	
Tuesday	Swim (Easy with drills)	0:30
Wednesday	Bike (Easy with drills)	0:30
Thursday	Run (Easy with drills)	0:30
Friday	Rest day	
Saturday	Run (20-min LT time trial)	0:45
Sunday	Swim (1,000-yd/m time trial)	0:45

Summary	Total	3:00
	Swim	1:15
	Bike	0:30
	Run	1:15

The Next Step

Depending upon the overall shape of your season, you can either repeat this training block or advance to the next one of the 4-part series.

If you repeat this training block, increase your training volume by approximately 10 percent and/or increase the time you spend at threshold pace.

When you advance to the next training block, adjust your first week's training volume so it is equal to or slightly below where you finished the third week of this one.

3 - Build Upon Your Base

Welcome to the build phase of your training. This 4-week training block provides you with a 3-up/1-down periodization schedule. You can change it to a 2-up/1-down schedule by simply deleting the third week.

The last week of the training block is a recovery week with testing scheduled at the end. The tests allow you to monitor your progress and (if needed) recalibrate your training zones.

Suggested distances/durations for each workout are provided; but you should adjust the weekly training volume so it equals what you did in the third week of the previous one.

Rearrange the workouts on your calendar as needed. Do so with an eye toward maintaining a consistent spacing between workouts of a particular discipline and balancing harder days with easier days.

Once you've completed this training block, you can move into your peak/race phase. About six weeks of higher intensity anaerobic training is usually sufficient in the lead-up to your target race or series of races; much more than that can lead to overtraining or mental fatigue. So, keep this in mind as you decide whether to repeat part of this training block before advancing to the next one in the 4-part series: the final peak/race phase.

Week 1 – Build Upon Your Base (2 Workouts/Discipline)

Monday	Rest day	
Tuesday	Swim (Fartlek 25s, drills)	0:40
	Strength (Shoulders/back)	0:20
Wednesday	Bike (Easy with short sprints)	0:50
Thursday	Run (Easy with striders, drills)	0:40
	Strength (Core/legs)	0:20
Friday	Swim (VO2 100s)	1:00
Saturday	Bike (VO2 intervals 3/2)	1:30
	or (VO2 intervals of 4/3 or 5/4)	
Sunday	Run (VO2 intervals 3/2)	1:00
	or (VO2 intervals of 4/3 or 5/4)	
Summary	Total 6:20	
	Swim 1:40	
	Bike 2:20	
	Run 1:40	
	Strength 0:40	

Week 2 – Build Upon Your Base (2 Workouts/Discipline)

Monday	Rest day	
Tuesday	Swim (Fartlek 25s, drills)	0:40
	Strength (Shoulders/back)	0:20
Wednesday	Bike (Easy with short sprints)	0:50
Thursday	Run (Easy with striders, drills)	0:40
	Strength (Core/legs)	0:20

Friday	Swim (VO2 200s)	1:00
Saturday	Bike (VO2 intervals 4/3) or (VO2 intervals of 3/2 or 5/4)	1:30
Sunday	Run (VO2 intervals 4/3) or (VO2 intervals of 3/2 or 5/4)	1:00
Summary	Total 6:20 Swim 1:40 Bike 2:20 Run 1:40 Strength 0:40	

Week 3 – Build Upon Your Base (2 Workouts/Discipline)

Monday	Rest day	
Tuesday	Swim (Fartlek 25s, drills) Strength (Shoulders/back)	0:40 0:20
Wednesday	Bike (Easy with short sprints)	0:50
Thursday	Run (Easy with striders, drills) Strength (Core/legs)	0:40 0:20
Friday	Swim (VO2 300s)	1:00
Saturday	Bike (VO2 intervals 5/4) or (VO2 intervals of 3/2 or 4/3)	1:30
Sunday	Run (VO2 intervals 5/4) or (VO2 intervals of 3/2 or 4/3)	1:00
Summary	Total 6:20 Swim 1:40 Bike 2:20 Run 1:40	

Strength   0:40

Week 4 – Recovery and Testing

Monday	Rest day	
Tuesday	Swim (Easy with drills)	0:30
Wednesday	Bike (Easy with drills)	0:30
Thursday	Run (Easy with drills)	0:30
Friday	Rest day	
Saturday	Run (20-min LT time trial)	0:45
Sunday	Swim (1,000-yd/m time trial)	0:45
Summary	Total 3:00 Swim 1:15 Bike 0:30 Run 1:15	

The Next Step

About six weeks of higher intensity anaerobic training is usually sufficient in the lead-up to your target race or series of races. Keep this in mind as you decide whether to repeat part of this training block before advancing to the next one.

If you repeat all or part of this training block, maintain or decrease the overall volume while increasing time at higher intensity (such as by increasing the number of intervals or interval work time).

4 – Peak for Your Race

Welcome to the peak racing phase of your season. This training block provides you with a 4-week plan to help you sharpen and taper for your peak race, and then recover from that race.

Keep in mind that everyone responds differently to a race taper. As you gain experience, you will learn what works best for you and you can adjust your plan accordingly.

Suggested distances/durations for each workout are provided; but you should adjust the weekly training volume so it equals what you did in the third week of the previous one.

Rearrange the workouts on your calendar as needed. Do so with an eye toward maintaining a consistent spacing between workouts of a particular discipline and balancing harder days with easier days.

The last week of this training block includes a post-race recovery week. Depending upon the length of your race and your state of recovery, you can repeat this recovery week more than once. Add/subtract workouts and durations as needed. The point is to do some easy activity to aid recovery and maintain fitness until you're ready to resume regular training.

Week 1 – Peak for Your Race (2 Workouts/Discipline)

Day	Workout	Duration
Monday	Rest day	
Tuesday	Swim (Fartlek 25s, drills)	0:40
	Strength (Shoulders/back)	0:20
Wednesday	Bike (Easy with short sprints)	0:50
Thursday	Run (Easy with striders, drills)	0:40
	Strength (Core/legs)	0:20
Friday	Swim (VO2 200s)	1:00
Saturday	Bike (VO2 intervals 4/3) or (VO2 intervals of 3/2 or 5/4)	1:30
Sunday	Run (VO2 intervals 3/2) or (VO2 intervals of 4/3 or 5/4)	1:00
Summary	Total 6:20	
	Swim 1:40	
	Bike 2:20	

Run	1:40	
Strength	0:40	

Week 2 – Peak for Your Race (2 Workouts/Discipline)

Monday	Rest day	
Tuesday	Swim (Easy with Drills)	0:30
Wednesday	Bike (Easy with drills)	0:45
Thursday	Run (Easy with striders, drills)	0:30
Friday	Swim (Fartlek 25s, drills)	0:40
Saturday	Bike (Sub-LT 20min tempo)	1:15
Sunday	Run (Sub-LT cruise intervals 8/2)	0:50
Summary	Total 4:30	
	Swim 1:10	
	Bike 2:00	
	Run 1:20	

Week 3 – Race Week

Monday	Rest day	
Tuesday	Swim (VO2 100s)	0:40
Wednesday	Bike (VO2 intervals 4/3)	1:00
Thursday	Run (VO2 intervals 3/2)	0:30
Friday	Rest day	
Saturday	Swim (Pre-race warmup)	0:10
	Bike (Pre-race warmup)	0:20
	Run (Pre-race warmup)	0:10

Sunday	Race day	
Summary	Total	2:50
	Swim	0:50
	Bike	1:20
	Run	0:40

Week 4 – Post-Race Recovery

Think active recovery this week. This means easy workouts interspersed with adequate rest. Take rest days as needed, but be sure to get out for some easy swimming, biking and/or running throughout the week to get the blood flowing and loosen up the muscles.

Monday	Swim (Easy)	0:20
Tuesday	Rest day	
Wednesday	Run (Easy)	0:30
Thursday	Bike (Easy)	0:45
Friday	Swim (Easy with drills)	0:30
Saturday	Bike (Easy with drills)	0:45
Sunday	Run (Easy with drills)	0:30
Summary	Total	3:20
	Swim	0:50
	Bike	1:30
	Run	1:00

The Next Step

Where you go from here depends on where you are in your season.

If you're in the middle of the season and your next A-level race occurs later in the year; return to a base building training block after one or two easy recovery weeks. Then build up from there to your target race or races at the end of the season.

If you have two or more A-level races in the upcoming weeks, maintain your peak fitness by doing race-level intensity workouts every two or three days. Ensure adequate recovery between those workouts. This is the time for maintaining or decreasing overall training volume while maintaining or increasing intensity to keep you both sharp and rested.

If you're at the end of your season; take a week off plus several unstructured easy weeks to refresh physically and mentally before beginning the new season with the first phase of base training.

3 Workouts/Discipline/Week

1 – Establish Your Base

Welcome to your first phase of base training. This 4-week training block provides you with a 3-up/1-down periodization schedule. You can change it to a 2-up/1-down schedule by simply deleting the third week.

The last week of the training block is a recovery week with testing scheduled at the end. The tests allow you to monitor your progress and (if needed) recalibrate your training zones.

Suggested distances/durations for each workout are provided; but you should adjust up or down according to your personal starting point.

Rearrange the workouts on your calendar as needed. Do so with an eye toward maintaining a consistent spacing between workouts of a particular discipline and balancing harder days with easier days.

This training block can be repeated multiple times early in the base training part of your season as you increase your training volume. As a rule of thumb, add about 10 percent to your training volume each time you repeat the training block.

Week 1 – Establish Your Base (3 Workouts/Discipline)

Monday	Rest day	
Tuesday	Swim (Easy with drills)	0:30
	Run (Easy with drills)	0:30
	Strength (Shoulders/back)	0:20
Wednesday	Swim (Fartlek 25s, drills)	0:40
	Bike (Easy with drills)	0:30
Thursday	BRICK (back-to-back bike/run)	
	Bike (Endurance with short sprints)	1:15
	Run (Endurance with striders)	0:45
Friday	Swim (Aerobic base 100s)	1:00
	Strength (Core/legs)	0:20
Saturday	Bike (Long)	1:45
Sunday	Run (Long)	1:00
Summary	Total	8:35
	Swim	2:10
	Bike	3:30
	Run	2:15
	Strength	0:40

Week 2 – Establish Your Base (3 Workouts/Discipline)

Monday	Rest day	
Tuesday	Swim (Easy with drills)	0:30
	Run (Easy with drills)	0:30
	Strength (Shoulders/back)	0:20
Wednesday	Swim (Fartlek 25s, drills)	0:40
	Bike (Easy with drills)	0:30

Thursday	BRICK (back-to-back bike/run)	
	Bike (Endurance with short sprints)	1:15
	Run (Endurance with striders)	0:45
Friday	Swim (Aerobic base 200s)	1:00
	Strength (Core/legs)	0:20
Saturday	Bike (Long)	2:00
Sunday	Run (Long)	1:15
Summary	Total 9:05	
	Swim 2:10	
	Bike 3:45	
	Run 2:30	
	Strength 0:40	

Week 3 – Establish Your Base (3 Workouts/Discipline)

Monday	Rest day	
Tuesday	Swim (Easy with drills)	0:30
	Run (Easy with drills)	0:30
	Strength (Shoulders/back)	0:20
Wednesday	Swim (Fartlek 25s, drills)	0:40
	Bike (Easy with drills)	0:30
Thursday	BRICK (back-to-back bike/run)	
	Bike (Endurance with short sprints)	1:15
	Run (Endurance with striders)	0:45
Friday	Swim (Aerobic base 500s)	1:00
	Strength (Core/legs)	0:20
Saturday	Bike (Long)	2:30
Sunday	Run (Long)	1:30

Summary	Total	9:50
	Swim	2:10
	Bike	4:15
	Run	2:45
	Strength	0:40

Week 4 – Recovery and Testing

Monday	Rest day	
Tuesday	Swim (Easy with drills)	0:30
	Bike (Endurance)	1:00
Wednesday	Run (Easy with drills)	0:30
Thursday	Bike (Easy with drills)	0:45
Friday	Rest day	
Saturday	Run (20-min LT time trial)	0:45
Sunday	Swim (1,000-yd/m time trial)	0:45
Summary	Total 4:15	
	Swim 1:15	
	Bike 1:45	
	Run 1:15	

The Next Step

Depending upon the overall shape of your season, you can either repeat this training block or advance to the next training block of the 4-step series.

If you repeat this training block, increase your training volume by approximately 10 percent. When you advance to the next block, adjust your first week's training volume so it is no more than 10 percent above where you finished the third week of this one.

2 – Develop Your Base

Welcome to your second phase of base training. This 4-week training block provides you with a 3-up/1-down periodization schedule. You can change it to a 2-up/1-down schedule by simply deleting the third week.

The last week of the training block is a recovery week with testing scheduled at the end. The tests allow you to monitor your progress and (if needed) recalibrate your training zones.

Suggested distances/durations for each workout are provided; but you should adjust the first week's training volume so it is no more than 10 percent above the third week's volume of the previous training block. From there, either maintain or slightly increase the volume of weeks two and three.

Rearrange the workouts on your calendar as needed. Do so with an eye toward maintaining a consistent spacing between workouts of a particular discipline and balancing harder days with easier days.

This training block can be repeated multiple times during the late base training part of your season as you increase your training volume and/or time spent at threshold pace.

Week 1 – Develop Your Base (3 Workouts/Discipline)

Day	Workout	Duration
Monday	Rest day	
Tuesday	Swim (Fartlek 25s, drills)	0:30
	Bike (Easy with short sprints)	0:30
	Strength (Core/legs)	0:20
Wednesday	Run (Sub-LT cruise intervals 8/2)	0:45
	Swim (Base tempo 100s)	0:45
Thursday	BRICK (back-to-back bike/run)	
	Bike (Sub-LT 20min tempo)	1:15
	Run (Easy with striders, drills)	0:30
Friday	Swim (Aerobic base 300s)	1:00
	Strength (Shoulders/back)	0:20

Saturday	Bike (Long)	2:30
Sunday	Run (Long)	1:30
Summary	Total 9:55 Swim 2:15 Bike 4:15 Run 2:45 Strength 0:40	

Week 2 – Develop Your Base (3 Workouts/Discipline)

Monday	Rest day	
Tuesday	Swim (Fartlek 25s, drills)	0:30
	Bike (Easy with short sprints)	0:30
	Strength (Core/legs)	0:20
Wednesday	Run (Sub-LT 20min tempo)	0:55
	Swim (LT cruise 300s)	0:45
Thursday	BRICK (back-to-back bike/run)	
	Bike (Sub-LT cruise intervals 8/2)	1:30
	Run (Easy with striders, drills)	0:30
Friday	Swim (Aerobic base 400s)	1:00
	Strength (Shoulders/back)	0:20
Saturday	Bike (Long)	2:30
Sunday	Run (Long)	1:30
Summary	Total 10:20 Swim 2:15 Bike 4:30 Run 2:55 Strength 0:40	

Week 3 – Develop Your Base (3 Workouts/Discipline)

Monday	Rest day	
Tuesday	Swim (Fartlek 25s, drills)	0:30
	Bike (Easy with short sprints)	0:45
	Strength (Core/legs)	0:20
Wednesday	Run (Sub-LT cruise intervals 8/2)	1:05
	or Run (Sub-LT 20min tempo)	
	Swim (LT cruise 500s)	0:45
Thursday	BRICK (back-to-back bike/run)	
	Bike (Sub-LT 20min tempo)	1:30
	or Bike (Sub-LT cruise intervals 8/2)	
	Run (Easy with striders, drills)	0:30
Friday	Swim (Aerobic base 600s)	1:00
	Strength (Shoulders/back)	0:20
Saturday	Bike (Long)	2:30
Sunday	Run (Long)	1:30
Summary	Total 10:45	
	Swim 2:15	
	Bike 4:45	
	Run 3:05	
	Strength 0:40	

Week 4 – Recovery and Testing

Monday	Rest day	
Tuesday	Swim (Easy with drills)	0:30
	Bike (Endurance)	1:00
Wednesday	Run (Easy with drills)	0:45

Thursday	Bike (Easy with drills)	1:00
Friday	Rest day	
Saturday	Run (20-min LT time trial)	0:45
Sunday	Swim (1,000-yd/m time trial)	0:45
Summary	Total 4:45 Swim 1:15 Bike 2:00 Run 1:30	

The Next Step

Depending upon the overall shape of your season, you can either repeat this training block or advance to the next one of the 4-part series.

If you repeat this training block, increase your training volume by approximately 10 percent and/or increase the time you spend at threshold pace.

When you advance to the next training block, adjust your first week's training volume so it is equal to or slightly below where you finished the third week of this one.

3 – Build Upon Your Base

Welcome to the build phase of your training. This 4-week training block provides you with a 3-up/1-down periodization schedule. You can change it to a 2-up/1-down schedule by simply deleting the third week.

The last week of the training block is a recovery week with testing scheduled at the end. The tests allow you to monitor your progress and (if needed) recalibrate your training zones.

Suggested distances/durations for each workout are provided; but you should adjust the weekly training volume so it equals what you did in the third week of the previous one.

Rearrange the workouts on your calendar as needed. Do so with an eye toward maintaining a consistent spacing between workouts of a particular discipline and balancing harder days with easier days.

Once you've completed this training block, you can move into your peak/race phase. About six weeks of higher intensity anaerobic training is usually sufficient in the lead-up to your target race or series of races; much more than that can lead to overtraining or mental fatigue. So, keep this in mind as you decide whether to repeat part of this training block before advancing to the next one in the 4-part series: the final peak/race phase.

Week 1 – Build Upon Your Base (3 Workouts/Discipline)

Day	Workout	Time
Monday	Rest day	
Tuesday	Swim (Fartlek 25s, drills)	0:30
	Bike (Easy with short sprints)	0:45
	Strength (Core/legs)	0:20
Wednesday	Run (VO2 intervals 3/2)	1:00
	Swim (VO2 100s)	0:45
Thursday	BRICK (back-to-back bike/run)	
	Bike (VO2 intervals 3/2)	1:30
	Run (Easy with striders, drills)	0:30
Friday	Swim (Aerobic base 200s)	1:00
	Strength (Shoulders/back)	0:20
Saturday	Bike (Long)	2:30
Sunday	Run (Long)	1:30
Summary	Total	10:40
	Swim	2:15
	Bike	4:45
	Run	3:00
	Strength	0:40

Week 2 – Build Upon Your Base (3 Workouts/Discipline)

Monday	Rest day	
Tuesday	Swim (Fartlek 25s, drills)	0:30
	Bike (Easy with short sprints)	0:45
	Strength (Core/legs)	0:20
Wednesday	Run (VO2 intervals 4/3)	1:00
	Swim (VO2 200s)	0:45
Thursday	BRICK (back-to-back bike/run)	
	Bike (VO2 intervals 4/3)	1:30
	Run (Easy with striders, drills)	0:30
Friday	Swim (Aerobic base 300s)	1:00
	Strength (Shoulders/back)	0:20
Saturday	Bike (Long)	2:30
Sunday	Run (Long)	1:30
Summary	Total	10:40
	Swim	2:15
	Bike	4:45
	Run	3:00
	Strength	0:40

Week 3 – Build Upon Your Base (3 Workouts/Discipline)

Monday	Rest day	
Tuesday	Swim (Fartlek 25s, drills)	0:30
	Bike (Easy with short sprints)	0:45
	Strength (Core/legs)	0:20
Wednesday	Run (VO2 intervals 5/4)	1:00
	Swim (VO2 300s)	0:45

Thursday	BRICK (back-to-back bike/run)	
	Bike (VO2 intervals 5/4)	1:30
	Run (Easy with striders, drills)	0:30
Friday	Swim (Aerobic base 500s)	1:00
	Strength (Shoulders/back)	0:20
Saturday	Bike (Long)	2:30
Sunday	Run (Long)	1:30
Summary	Total 10:40	
	Swim 2:15	
	Bike 4:45	
	Run 3:00	
	Strength 0:40	

Week 4 – Recovery and Testing

Monday	Rest day	
Tuesday	Swim (Easy with drills)	0:30
	Bike (Endurance)	1:00
Wednesday	Run (Easy with drills)	0:45
Thursday	Bike (Easy with drills)	1:00
Friday	Rest day	
Saturday	Run (20-min LT time trial)	0:45
Sunday	Swim (1,000-yd/m time trial)	0:45
Summary	Total 4:45	
	Swim 1:15	
	Bike 2:00	
	Run 1:30	

The Next Step

About six weeks of higher intensity anaerobic training is usually sufficient in the lead-up to your target race or series of races. Keep this in mind as you decide whether to repeat part of this training block before advancing to the next one.

If you repeat all or part of this training block, maintain or decrease the overall volume while increasing time at higher intensity (such as by increasing the number of intervals or interval work time).

4 – Peak for Your Race

Welcome to the peak racing phase of your season. This training block provides you with a 4-week plan to help you sharpen and taper for your peak race, and then recover from that race.

Keep in mind that everyone responds differently to a race taper. As you gain experience, you will learn what works best for you and you can adjust your plan accordingly.

Suggested distances/durations for each workout are provided; but you should adjust the weekly training volume so it equals what you did in the third week of the previous one.

Rearrange the workouts on your calendar as needed. Do so with an eye toward maintaining a consistent spacing between workouts of a particular discipline and balancing harder days with easier days.

The last week of this training block includes a post-race recovery week. Depending upon the length of your race and your state of recovery, you can repeat this recovery week more than once. Add/subtract workouts and durations as needed. The point is to do some easy activity to aid recovery and maintain fitness until you you're ready to resume regular training.

Week 1 – Peak for Your Race (3 Workouts/Discipline)

Monday	Rest day	
Tuesday	Swim (Fartlek 25s, drills)	0:30
	Bike (Easy with short sprints)	0:45

	Strength (Core/legs)	0:20
Wednesday	Run (VO2 intervals 3/2)	1:00
	Swim (VO2 200s)	0:45
Thursday	BRICK (back-to-back bike/run)	
	Bike (VO2 intervals 4/3)	1:30
	Run (Easy with striders, drills)	0:30
Friday	Swim (Aerobic base 600s)	1:00
	Strength (Shoulders/back)	0:20
Saturday	Bike (Long)	2:30
Sunday	Run (Long)	1:30
Summary	Total 10:40	
	Swim 2:15	
	Bike 4:45	
	Run 3:00	
	Strength 0:40	

Week 2 – Peak for Your Race (3 Workouts/Discipline)

Monday	Rest day	
Tuesday	Swim (VO2 200s)	0:30
	Bike (Easy with short sprints)	0:30
Wednesday	Run (VO2 intervals 3/2)	0:45
	Swim (Fartlek 25s, drills)	0:30
Thursday	Bike (VO2 intervals 4/3)	1:00
	Run (Easy with striders, drills)	0:30
Friday	Swim (VO2 100s)	0:45
Saturday	Bike (Sub-LT 20min tempo)	1:15

Sunday	Run (Sub-LT cruise intervals 8/2)		0:45
Summary	Total	6:30	
	Swim	1:45	
	Bike	2:45	
	Run	2:00	

Week 3 – Race Week

Monday	Rest day	
Tuesday	Swim (VO2 100s)	0:30
	Bike (Easy)	0:20
Wednesday	Bike (VO2 intervals 3/2)	0:30
	Swim (Easy)	0:20
Thursday	Bike (VO2 intervals 4/3)	1:00
	Run (Easy)	0:20
Friday	Rest day	
Saturday	Swim (Pre-race warmup)	0:10
	Bike (Pre-race warmup)	0:20
	Run (Pre-race warmup)	0:10
Sunday	Race day	
Summary	Total	3:40
	Swim	1:00
	Bike	1:40
	Run	1:00

Week 4 – Post-Race Recovery

Think active recovery this week. This means easy workouts interspersed with adequate rest. Take rest days as needed, but be sure to get out for some easy swimming, biking and/or running throughout the week to get the blood flowing and loosen up the muscles.

Monday	Swim (Easy)	0:20
Tuesday	Rest day	
Wednesday	Run (Easy)	0:30
	Swim (Easy)	0:20
Thursday	Bike (Easy)	0:45
	Run (Easy)	0:20
Friday	Swim (Easy with drills)	0:30
Saturday	Bike (Easy with drills)	0:45
Sunday	Run (Easy with drills)	0:30
	Bike (Easy)	0:30
Summary	Total 4:30	
	Swim 1:10	
	Bike 2:00	
	Run 1:20	

The Next Step

Where you go from here depends on where you are in your season.

If you're in the middle of the season and your next A-level race occurs later in the year; return to a base building training block after one or two easy recovery weeks. Then build up from there to your target race or races at the end of the season.

If you have two or more A-level races in the upcoming weeks, maintain your peak fitness by doing race-level intensity workouts every two or three days. Ensure adequate recovery between those workouts. This is the time for maintaining or decreasing overall training volume while maintaining or increasing intensity to keep you both sharp and rested.

If you're at the end of your season; take a week off plus several unstructured easy weeks to refresh physically and mentally before beginning the new season with the first phase of base training.

4 Workouts/Discipline/Week

1 – Establish Your Base

Welcome to your first phase of base training. This 4-week training block provides you with a 3-up/1-down periodization schedule. You can change it to a 2-up/1-down schedule by simply deleting the third week.

The last week of the training block is a recovery week with testing scheduled at the end. The tests allow you to monitor your progress and (if needed) recalibrate your training zones.

Suggested distances/durations for each workout are provided; but you should adjust up or down according to your personal starting point.

Rearrange the workouts on your calendar as needed. Do so with an eye toward maintaining a consistent spacing between workouts of a particular discipline and balancing harder days with easier days.

This training block can be repeated multiple times early in the base training part of your season as you increase your training volume. As a rule of thumb, add about 10 percent to your training volume each time you repeat the training block.

Week 1 – Establish Your Base (4 Workouts/Discipline)

Monday	Swim (Easy with drills)	0:30
Tuesday	Swim (Fartlek 25s, drills)	0:40
	Bike (Endurance with short sprints)	1:15
	Strength (Shoulders/back)	0:20
Wednesday	BRICK (back-to-back bike/run)	
	Bike (Endurance)	1:15
	Run (Endurance)	0:45
	Swim (Aerobic base 100s)	0:45

Thursday	Run (Endurance with striders)	0:45
	Bike (Easy with drills)	0:30
	Strength (Core/legs)	0:20
Friday	Swim (Aerobic base 500s)	1:00
	Run (Easy with drills)	0:30
Saturday	Bike (Long)	1:45
Sunday	Run (Long)	1:00
Summary	Total 11:20	
	Swim 2:55	
	Bike 4:45	
	Run 3:00	
	Strength 0:40	

Week 2 – Establish Your Base (4 Workouts/Discipline)

Monday	Swim (Easy with drills)	0:30
Tuesday	Swim (Fartlek 25s, drills)	0:40
	Bike (Endurance with short sprints)	1:15
	Strength (Shoulders/back)	0:20
Wednesday	BRICK (back-to-back bike/run)	
	Bike (Endurance)	1:15
	Run (Endurance)	0:45
	Swim (Aerobic base 100s)	0:45
Thursday	Run (Endurance with striders)	0:45
	Bike (Easy with drills)	0:30
	Strength (Core/legs)	0:20
Friday	Swim (Aerobic base 500s)	1:00
	Run (Easy with drills)	0:30
Saturday	Bike (Long)	2:00

Sunday	Run (Long)		1:15
Summary	Total	11:50	
	Swim	2:55	
	Bike	5:00	
	Run	3:15	
	Strength	0:40	

Week 3 – Establish Your Base (4 Workouts/Discipline)

Monday	Swim (Easy with drills)		0:30
Tuesday	Swim (Fartlek 25s, drills)		0:40
	Bike (Endurance with short sprints)		1:15
	Strength (Shoulders/back)		0:20
Wednesday	BRICK (back-to-back bike/run)		
	Bike (Endurance)		1:15
	Run (Endurance)		0:45
	Swim (Aerobic base 100s)		0:45
Thursday	Run (Endurance with striders)		0:45
	Bike (Easy with drills)		0:30
	Strength (Core/legs)		0:20
Friday	Swim (Aerobic base 500s)		1:00
	Run (Easy with drills)		0:30
Saturday	Bike (Long)		2:30
Sunday	Run (Long)		1:30
Summary	Total	12:35	
	Swim	2:55	
	Bike	5:30	
	Run	3:30	
	Strength	0:40	

Week 4 – Recovery and Testing

Monday	Swim (Easy with drills)	0:30
Tuesday	Run (Endurance)	0:30
	Bike (Easy with drills)	1:00
Wednesday	Swim (Aerobic base 100s)	0:45
	Bike (Endurance)	1:00
Thursday	Run (Easy with drills)	0:30
	Bike (Easy)	0:30
Friday	Rest day	
Saturday	Run (20-min LT time trial)	0:45
Sunday	Swim (1,000-yd/m time trial)	0:45
Summary	Total 5:45	
	Swim 2:00	
	Bike 2:00	
	Run 1:45	

The Next Step

Depending upon the overall shape of your season, you can either repeat this training block or advance to the next training block of the 4-step series.

If you repeat this training block, increase your training volume by approximately 10 percent. When you advance to the next block, adjust your first week's training volume so it is no more than 10 percent above where you finished the third week of this one.percent above where you finished the third week of this module.

2 – Develop Your Base

Welcome to your second phase of base training. This 4-week

training block provides you with a 3-up/1-down periodization schedule. You can change it to a 2-up/1-down schedule by simply deleting the third week.

The last week of the training block is a recovery week with testing scheduled at the end. The tests allow you to monitor your progress and (if needed) recalibrate your training zones.

Suggested distances/durations for each workout are provided; but you should adjust the first week's training volume so it is no more than 10 percent above the third week's volume of the previous training block. From there, either maintain or slightly increase the volume of weeks two and three.

Rearrange the workouts on your calendar as needed. Do so with an eye toward maintaining a consistent spacing between workouts of a particular discipline and balancing harder days with easier days.

This training block can be repeated multiple times during the late base training part of your season as you increase your training volume and/or time spent at threshold pace.

Week 1 – Develop Your Base (4 Workouts/Discipline)

Day	Workout	Duration
Monday	Swim (Easy with drills)	0:30
Tuesday	Swim (Fartlek 25s, drills)	0:30
	Bike (Endurance)	1:30
	Run (Easy with drills, striders)	0:30
Wednesday	Run (Sub-LT cruise intervals 8/2)	1:00
	Bike (Easy with short sprints)	0:30
	Strength (Core/legs)	0:20
Thursday	Swim (Base tempo 100s)	0:45
	BRICK (back-to-back bike/run)	
	Bike (Sub-LT 20min tempo)	1:15
	Run (Endurance)	0:45
Friday	Swim (Aerobic base 300s)	1:00
	Strength (Shoulders/back)	0:20
Saturday	Bike (Long)	2:30

Sunday	Run (Long)		1:30
Summary	Total	13:10	
	Swim	2:45	
	Bike	6:00	
	Run	3:45	
	Strength	0:40	

Week 2 – Develop Your Base (4 Workouts/Discipline)

Monday	Swim (Easy with drills)	0:30
Tuesday	Swim (Fartlek 25s, drills)	0:30
	Bike (Endurance)	1:45
	Run (Easy with drills, striders)	0:30
Wednesday	Run (Sub-LT 20min tempo)	1:10
	Bike (Easy with short sprints)	0:30
	Strength (Core/legs)	0:20
Thursday	Swim (LT Cruise 300s)	0:45
	BRICK (back-to-back bike/run)	
	Bike (Sub-LT cruise intervals 8/2)	1:30
	Run (Endurance)	0:45
Friday	Swim (Aerobic base 400s)	1:00
	Strength (Shoulders/back)	0:20
Saturday	Bike (Long)	2:30
Sunday	Run (Long)	1:30

Summary	Total	13:35
	Swim	2:45
	Bike	6:15
	Run	3:55
	Strength	0:40

Week 3 – Develop Your Base (4 Workouts/Discipline)

Monday	Swim (Easy with drills)	0:30
Tuesday	Swim (Fartlek 25s, drills)	0:30
	Bike (Endurance)	2:00
	Run (Easy with drills, striders)	0:30
Wednesday	Run (Sub-LT cruise intervals 8/2) or Run (Sub-LT 20min tempo)	1:20
	Bike (Easy with short sprints)	0:30
	Strength (Core/legs)	0:20
Thursday	Swim (LT Cruise 500s)	0:45
	BRICK (back-to-back bike/run)	
	Bike (Sub-LT 20min tempo) or (Sub-LT cruise intervals 8/2)	1:30
	Run (Endurance)	0:45
Friday	Swim (Aerobic base 600s)	1:00
	Strength (Shoulders/back)	0:20
Saturday	Bike (Long)	2:30
Sunday	Run (Long)	1:30
Summary	Total 14:00	
	Swim 2:45	
	Bike 6:30	
	Run 4:05	
	Strength 0:40	

Week 4 – Recovery and Testing

Monday	Swim (Easy with drills)	0:30
Tuesday	Run (Endurance)	0:30
	Bike (Easy with drills)	0:30

Wednesday	Swim (Aerobic base 100s)	0:45
	Bike (Endurance)	1:00
Thursday	Run (Easy with drills)	0:45
	Bike (Easy)	0:45
Friday	Rest day	
Saturday	Run (20-min LT time trial)	0:45
Sunday	Swim (1,000-yd/m time trial)	0:45
Summary	Total 6:15	
	Swim 2:00	
	Bike 2:15	
	Run 2:00	

The Next Step

Depending upon the overall shape of your season, you can either repeat this training block or advance to the next one of the 4-part series.

If you repeat this training block, increase your training volume by approximately 10 percent and/or increase the time you spend at threshold pace.

When you advance to the next training block, adjust your first week's training volume so it is equal to or slightly below where you finished the third week of this one.

3 – Build Upon Your Base

Welcome to the build phase of your training. This 4-week training block provides you with a 3-up/1-down periodization schedule. You can change it to a 2-up/1-down schedule by simply deleting the third week.

The last week of the training block is a recovery week with testing scheduled at the end. The tests allow you to monitor your progress and (if needed) recalibrate your training zones.

Suggested distances/durations for each workout are provided; but you should adjust the weekly training volume so it equals what you did in the third week of the previous one.

Rearrange the workouts on your calendar as needed. Do so with an eye toward maintaining a consistent spacing between workouts of a particular discipline and balancing harder days with easier days.

Once you've completed this training block, you can move into your peak/race phase. About six weeks of higher intensity anaerobic training is usually sufficient in the lead-up to your target race or series of races; much more than that can lead to overtraining or mental fatigue. So, keep this in mind as you decide whether to repeat part of this training block before advancing to the next one in the 4-part series: the final peak/race phase.

Week 1 – Build Upon Your Base (4 Workouts/Discipline)

Day	Workout	Duration
Monday	Swim (Easy with drills)	0:30
Tuesday	Swim (Fartlek 25s, drills)	0:30
	Bike (Endurance)	2:00
	Run (Easy with drills, striders)	0:30
Wednesday	Run (VO2 intervals 3/2)	1:00
	Bike (Easy with short sprints)	0:30
	Strength (Core/legs)	0:20
Thursday	Swim (VO2 100s)	0:45
	BRICK (back-to-back bike/run)	
	Bike (VO2 intervals 3/2)	1:30
	Run (Endurance)	0:45
Friday	Swim (Aerobic base 200s)	1:00
	Strength (Shoulders/back)	0:20
Saturday	Bike (Long)	2:30
Sunday	Run (Long)	1:30
Summary	Total	13:40

Swim	2:45
Bike	6:30
Run	3:45
Strength	0:40

Week 2 – Build Upon Your Base (4 Workouts/Discipline)

Monday	Swim (Easy with drills)	0:30
Tuesday	Swim (Fartlek 25s, drills)	0:30
	Bike (Endurance)	2:00
	Run (Easy with drills, striders)	0:30
Wednesday	Run (VO2 intervals 4/3)	1:00
	Bike (Easy with short sprints)	0:30
	Strength (Core/legs)	0:20
Thursday	Swim (VO2 200s)	0:45
	BRICK (back-to-back bike/run)	
	Bike (VO2 intervals 4/3)	1:30
	Run (Endurance)	0:45
Friday	Swim (Aerobic base 300s)	1:00
	Strength (Shoulders/back)	0:20
Saturday	Bike (Long)	2:30
Sunday	Run (Long)	1:30
Summary	Total 13:40	
	Swim 2:45	
	Bike 6:30	
	Run 3:45	
	Strength 0:40	

Week 3 – Build Upon Your Base (4 Workouts/Discipline)

Monday	Swim (Easy with drills)	0:30

Tuesday	Swim (Fartlek 25s, drills)	0:30
	Bike (Endurance)	2:00
	Run (Easy with drills, striders)	0:30
Wednesday	Run (VO2 intervals 5/4)	1:00
	Bike (Easy with short sprints)	0:30
	Strength (Core/legs)	0:20
Thursday	Swim (VO2 300s)	0:45
	BRICK (back-to-back bike/run)	
	Bike (VO2 intervals 5/4)	1:30
	Run (Endurance)	0:45
Friday	Swim (Aerobic base 500s)	1:00
	Strength (Shoulders/back)	0:20
Saturday	Bike (Long)	2:30
Sunday	Run (Long)	1:30
Summary	Total	13:40
	Swim	2:45
	Bike	6:30
	Run	3:45
	Strength	0:40

Week 4 – Recovery and Testing

Monday	Swim (Easy with drills)	0:30
Tuesday	Run (Endurance)	0:30
	Bike (Easy with drills)	0:30
Wednesday	Swim (Aerobic base 100s)	0:45
	Bike (Endurance)	1:00
Thursday	Run (Easy with drills)	0:45
	Bike (Easy)	0:45

Friday	Rest day	
Saturday	Run (20-min LT time trial)	0:45
Sunday	Swim (1,000-yd/m time trial)	0:45
Summary	Total 6:15 Swim 2:00 Bike 2:15 Run 2:00	

The Next Step

About six weeks of higher intensity anaerobic training is usually sufficient in the lead-up to your target race or series of races. Keep this in mind as you decide whether to repeat part of this training block before advancing to the next one.

If you repeat all or part of this training block, maintain or decrease the overall volume while increasing time at higher intensity (such as by increasing the number of intervals or interval work time).

4 – Peak for Your Race

Welcome to the peak racing phase of your season. This training block provides you with a 4-week plan to help you sharpen and taper for your peak race, and then recover from that race.

Keep in mind that everyone responds differently to a race taper. As you gain experience, you will learn what works best for you and you can adjust your plan accordingly.

Suggested distances/durations for each workout are provided; but you should adjust the weekly training volume so it equals what you did in the third week of the previous one.

Rearrange the workouts on your calendar as needed. Do so with an eye toward maintaining a consistent spacing between workouts of a particular discipline and balancing harder days with easier days.

The last week of this training block includes a post-race recovery week. Depending upon the length of your race and your state of recovery, you can repeat this recovery week more than once.

Add/subtract workouts and durations as needed. The point is to do some easy activity to aid recovery and maintain fitness until you you're ready to resume regular training.

Week 1 – Peak for Your Race (4 Workouts/Discipline)

Monday	Swim (Easy with drills)	0:30
Tuesday	Swim (Fartlek 25s, drills)	0:30
	Bike (Endurance)	2:00
	Run (Easy with drills, striders)	0:30
Wednesday	Run (VO2 intervals 3/2)	1:00
	Bike (Easy with short sprints)	0:30
	Strength (Core/legs)	0:20
Thursday	Swim (VO2 200s)	0:45
	BRICK (back-to-back bike/run)	
	Bike (VO2 intervals 4/3)	1:30
	Run (Endurance)	0:45
Friday	Swim (Aerobic base 600s)	1:00
	Strength (Shoulders/back)	0:20
Saturday	Bike (Long)	2:30
Sunday	Run (Long)	1:30
Summary	Total	13:40
	Swim	2:45
	Bike	6:30
	Run	3:45
	Strength	0:40

Week 2 – Peak for Your Race (4 Workouts/Discipline)

Monday	Swim (Easy with drills)	0:30

Tuesday	Swim (VO2 200s)	0:30
	Bike (Easy with short sprints)	0:30
	Run (Easy)	0:20
Wednesday	Run (VO2 intervals 3/2)	0:45
	Swim (Fartlek 25s, drills)	0:30
	Bike (Easy)	0:20
Thursday	Bike (VO2 intervals 4/3)	1:00
	Run (Easy with striders, drills)	0:30
Friday	Swim (VO2 100s)	0:45
Saturday	Bike (Sub-LT 20min tempo)	1:15
Sunday	Run (Sub-LT cruise intervals 8/2)	0:45
Summary	Total 7:40	
	Swim 2:15	
	Bike 3:05	
	Run 2:20	

Week 3 – Race Week

Monday	Rest day	
Tuesday	Swim (VO2 100s)	0:30
	Bike (Easy)	0:20
Wednesday	Bike (VO2 intervals 3/2)	0:30
	Swim (Easy)	0:20
Thursday	Bike (VO2 intervals 4/3)	1:00
	Run (Easy)	0:20
Friday	Rest day	
Saturday	Swim (Pre-race warmup)	0:10
	Bike (Pre-race warmup)	0:20

	Run (Pre-race warmup)	0:10
Sunday	Race day	
Summary	Total 3:40 Swim 1:00 Bike 1:40 Run 1:00	

Week 4 – Post-Race Recovery

Think active recovery this week. This means easy workouts interspersed with adequate rest. Take rest days as needed, but be sure to get out for some easy swimming, biking and/or running throughout the week to get the blood flowing and loosen up the muscles.

Monday	Swim (Easy)	0:20
Tuesday	Rest day	
Wednesday	Run (Easy) Bike (Easy) Swim (Easy)	0:20 0:20 0:20
Thursday	Bike (Easy) Run (Easy)	0:20 0:20
Friday	Run (Easy) Swim (Easy with drills)	0:20 0:30
Saturday	Bike (Easy with drills) Swim (Easy with drills)	0:30 0:30
Sunday	Run (Easy with drills) Bike (Easy)	0:30 0:30
Summary	Total 4:50 Swim 1:40 Bike 1:40	

Run   1:30

The Next Step

Where you go from here depends on where you are in your season.

If you're in the middle of the season and your next A-level race occurs later in the year; return to a base building training block after one or two easy recovery weeks. Then build up from there to your target race or races at the end of the season.

If you have two or more A-level races in the upcoming weeks, maintain your peak fitness by doing race-level intensity workouts every two or three days. Ensure adequate recovery between those workouts. This is the time for maintaining or decreasing overall training volume while maintaining or increasing intensity to keep you both sharp and rested.

If you're at the end of your season; take a week off plus several unstructured easy weeks to refresh physically and mentally before beginning the new season with the first phase of base training.

9
Swim Workouts

Recovery Workouts

Swim (Easy with Optional Drills)

When: All training phases, especially base training

Why: To aid recovery, add to your training volume and loosen you up for the key workouts of the week

What: Swim in Zone 1 or at an "easy" pace. Optional: incorporate drills into the swim.

Where: Pool or open water

How: Use perceived exertion or pace to monitor intensity

Swim (Form – Beginner Workout 1)

When: All training phases, especially base training

Why: To develop proper form and efficient mechanics while adding to your training volume

What: 4 x 25 count strokes per length with rest as needed. Record these numbers so you know your average. If your number is above 20 strokes per 25 yards; your aim is to eventually lower that below 20. (Note: one arm equals one 'stroke.')

12 x 25 "swimming downhill" with rest as needed. To get

the sensation of "swimming downhill," think of your chest/lungs as a big buoy (like an inflatable beach ball) that you want to push down into the water. Press this buoy (your chest) into the water, and let the force of the water pushing back raise your hips and legs to the surface.

6 x 50 swimming with a "weightless arm" with 10-20 seconds rest interval. As you extend your arm forward during entry, imagine that arm being weightless. In other words, you don't want it to sink or fight against the water by letting it drop straight down. If you find this difficult, remember to "press your buoy" and imagine you are reaching toward the wall at the end of the pool as if it were your last stroke.

12 x 25 rotating kick. Start off lying on one side with your bottom arm extended above your head and your top arm at your side. Kick about six times; then take a stroke and rotate to the other side. Repeat, rolling from side to side every six kicks or so. Aim to keep your body long and level as you rotate along the spine.

Warm down: 100 non-free (Total: 1500)

Where: Pool

How: Use perceived exertion to monitor intensity; don't worry about time

Swim (Form – Beginner Workout 2)

When: All training phases, especially base training

Why: To develop proper form and efficient mechanics while adding to your training volume

What: Warm up: 300 swim, 100 kick

4 x 25 count strokes per length with rest as needed. Once you know your average, subtract 2-4. This is your target number for the next set.

8 x 25 count strokes per length with rest as needed. The aim is to hit your target number without adding any additional beats to your kick. This should be challenging, but attainable on most of these 25s. Focus on making your body long and "slippery" through the water, like a long, narrow racing boat.

8 x 25 "front quadrant" swimming with rest as needed. Here, "quadrant" refers to the following. The water line represents the x-axis and a vertical line drawn through the shoulders represents the y-axis. As these lines intersect, they divide the space into four quadrants. Your aim in this set is to always have an arm extended in the "front quadrant" in front of the shoulder and under the water. In other words, once your front arm extends forward at entry, pause it in that position until your opposite arm finishes its stroke and enters into the front quadrant space.

12 x 50 (25 catch-up drill, 25 regular free) with 20 seconds rest interval. For the catch-up drill, keep your non-stroking arm extended in the front quadrant entry position until the opposite arm "catches up" to the same position. This slows down the stroke, emphasizes the pause after the forward extension upon entry, and exaggerates the "front quadrant" swimming.

8 x 25 rotating kick. Start off lying on one side with your bottom arm extended above your head and your top arm at your side. Kick about six times; then take a stroke and rotate to the other side. Repeat, rolling from side to side every six kicks or so. Aim to keep your body long and level as you rotate along the spine.

Warm down: 100 non-free (preferably backstroke)
(Total: 1500)

Where: Pool

How: Use perceived exertion to monitor intensity; don't worry about time

Swim (Form – Beginner Workout 3)

When: All training phases, especially base training

Why: To develop proper form and efficient mechanics while adding to your training volume

What: Warm up: 300 swim, 100 kick

4 x 100 free with rest as needed. For each 100 visualize a different aspect of form. #1 swim downhill by pressing the buoy. #2 make sure you are doing front quadrant swimming. #3 swim with a weightless arm. #4 any of the above as needed.

4 x 25 count strokes per length with rest as needed. Take your average stroke count and use this as your target number for the next set.

20 x 25 "stroke eliminators" with 15-20 rest interval. Start with a slow 25 at your target strokes per length from above. Note the time it takes to swim this. On the next 25, try to lower the time a bit while maintaining the same stroke count. Continue this pattern by going a little faster on each 25 until you can no longer maintain the target stroke count. At this point, slow down the time and maintain the stroke count.

Warm down: 100 non-free (preferably backstroke)

(Total: 1500)

Notes:
To get the sensation of "swimming downhill," think of your chest/lungs as a big buoy (like an inflatable beach ball) that you need to push down into the water. Press this buoy (your chest) into the water, and let the force of the water pushing back raise your hips and legs to the surface.

"Quadrant" refers to the following. The water line represents the x-axis and a vertical line drawn through the shoulders represents the y-axis. As these lines intersect, they divide the space into four quadrants. Your aim in this set is to always have an arm extended in the "front quadrant" in front of the shoulder and under the water. In other words, once your front arm extends forward at entry, pause it in that position until your opposite arm finishes its stroke and enters into the front quadrant space.

As you extend your arm forward during entry, imagine that arm being weightless. In other words, you don't want it to sink or fight against by letting it drop straight down. If you find this difficult, remember to "press your buoy" and imagine you are reaching toward the wall at the end of the pool as if it were your last stroke.

Where: Pool

How: Use perceived exertion to monitor intensity; don't worry about time

Swim (Form – Advanced Workout 1)

When: All training phases, especially base training

Why: To develop proper form and efficient mechanics while adding to your training volume

What: Warm up: 400 free, 200 non-free and/or kick

Set #1: 4-8 x 50 (25 fist drill, 25 regular free) Focus on keeping the elbow high and finding the most effective position for your arm during the pull phase of your stroke. Rest interval: 10-20 seconds. (200-400)

Set #2: 8-12 x 25 free (for form not speed; count strokes and aim to lower stroke count on these). Rest interval: as needed (e.g. 15-30 seconds). (200-300)

Set #3: 6-8 x 50 (25 rotating kick, 25 build [build speed to sprint]). Rest interval: 20 seconds. (300-400)

Warm down: 100 backstroke, 100 free, 100 choice.

(Total: 1500-2000)

Where: Pool

How: Use perceived exertion to monitor intensity; don't worry about time

Swim (Form – Advanced Workout 2)

When: All training phases, especially base training

Why: To develop proper form and efficient mechanics while adding to your training volume

What: Warm up: 400 free, 200 non-free and/or kick

Set #1: 4-8 x 75 (25 left-arm, 25 right-arm, 25 full stroke). Rest interval: 15-30 seconds. (300-600)

Set #2: 4-6 x 50 kick (25 kick on back, 25 rotating kick). Rest interval: 15-30 seconds. (200-300)

Set #3: 8 x 25 build (build speed to sprint). Recovery: 25 easy backstroke plus 5-10 seconds rest. (400)

Warmdown: 200 easy

(Total: 1700-2000)

Where: Pool

How: Use perceived exertion to monitor intensity; don't worry about time

Swim (Form – Advanced Workout 3)

When: All training phases, especially base training

Why: To develop proper form and efficient mechanics while adding to your training volume

What: Warm up: 400 free, 200 non-free and/or kick

Set #1: 4-6 x 100 (25 left-arm, 25 right-arm, 25 catch-up drill, 25 full stroke). Rest interval: 15-30 seconds. (400-600)

Set #2: 8-12 x 25 kick (odd 25s kick on back, even 25s rotating kick). Rest interval: 15-30 seconds. (200-300)

Set #3: 300-500 pull (work on breathing to both sides every three strokes; every fourth 25 fist drill)

Warmdown: 200 easy

(Total: 1700-2200)

Where: Pool

How: Use perceived exertion to monitor intensity; don't worry about time

Swim (Form – Advanced Workout 1 for Long Course)

When: All training phases, especially base training

Why: To develop proper form and efficient mechanics while adding to your training volume

What: Warm up: 400 free, 200 non-free and/or kick

Set #1: 4-8 x 50 (alternate 50 fist drill, 50 regular free). Focus on keeping the elbow high and finding the most effective position for your arm during the pull phase of your stroke. Rest interval: 10-20 seconds. (200-400)

Set #2: 4-6 x 50 free (for form not speed; count strokes and aim to lower stroke count on these). Rest interval: as needed (e.g. 15-30 seconds). (200-300)

Set #3: 6-8 x 50 (25 rotating kick, 25 build [build speed to sprint]). Rest interval: 20 seconds. (300-400)

Warm down: 100 backstroke, 100 free, 100 choice.

(Total: 1500-2,000)

Where: Pool (long course)

How: Use perceived exertion to monitor intensity; don't worry about time

Swim (Form – Advanced Workout 2 for Long Course)

When: All training phases, especially base training

Why: To develop proper form and efficient mechanics while adding to your training volume

What: Warm up: 400 free, 200 non-free and/or kick

Set #1: 3-6 x 100 (25 left-arm, 25 right-arm, 25 weakest arm, 25 full stroke). Rest interval: 15-30 seconds. (300-600)

Set #2: 4-6 x 50 kick (25 kick on back, 25 rotating kick). Rest interval: 15-30 seconds. (200-300)

Set #3: 8 x 25 build (build speed to sprint) w/25 easy backstroke recovery. Rest interval (after 50): 15-30 seconds. (400)

Warmdown: 200 easy

(Total: 1700-2000)

Where: Pool (long course)

How: Use perceived exertion to monitor intensity; don't worry about time

Swim (Form – Advanced Workout 3 for Long Course)

When: All training phases, especially base training

Why: To develop proper form and efficient mechanics while adding to your training volume

What:	Warm up: 400 free, 200 non-free and/or kick

          Set #1: 4-6 x 100 (25 left-arm, 25 right-arm, 25 catch-up drill, 25 full stroke). Rest interval: 15-30 seconds. (400-600)

          Set #2: 4-6 x 50 kick (odd 50s kick on back, even 50s rotating kick). Rest interval: 15-30 seconds. (200-300)

          Set #3: 300-500 pull (work on breathing to both sides every three strokes; every fourth 25 fist drill)

          Warmdown: 200 easy

          (Total: 1700-2200)

Where:	Pool (long course)
How:	Use perceived exertion to monitor intensity; don't worry about time

Swim (Freestyle Golf)

When:	All training phases, especially base training
Why:	To develop proper form and efficient mechanics while adding to your training volume
What:	Warm up: 400 free, 200 non-free and/or kick

          Set #1: 6-10 x 50 freestyle "golf" (a.k.a. "swolf"). Time the 50 and count your strokes. Add the two numbers together to get your score. (Some training devices do this for you automatically.) Aim to lower your score by increasing speed and/or decreasing your stroke count. For example, if you swim the 50 in 40 seconds and take 32 strokes, your score is 72. Rest interval: as needed (e.g. 15-30 seconds).

          Set #2: 300 pull

          Warm down: 200 easy backstroke
          (Total: 1400-2000)

Where: Pool (long course)

How: Use perceived exertion and pace to monitor intensity

Swim (Pre-race Warmup)

When: Day before a race

Why: To loosen up, check equipment, and scout out the course

What: This is effectively an "active rest day." Your aim is get in a short swim on the race course to check equipment and loosen up.

You will have a lot of energy, especially with the excitement of race week. But remember that today is not the race nor is it a day for an extended workout. Do just enough to get the blood flowing, keeping it in Zone 1 with a few short sprints.

Be sure to scout out where you want to line up for the start on race day. Stay hydrated and fueled. Eat well, and relax in preparation for the race.

Where: Race course (if possible)

How: Use perceived exertion and pace to monitor intensity

Endurance Workouts

Swim (Endurance)

When: All training phases, especially base training

Why: To build the aerobic base by developing the ability to better metabolize fat and spare glycogen (stored carbohydrate) as a long duration energy source

What: Swim primarily freestyle in Zone 2 or at a "conversational" pace. Incorporate drills and alternate strokes as desired.

Where: Pool or open water

How: Use perceived exertion or pace to monitor intensity

Swim (Fartlek in Pool)

When: All training phases, especially base training

Why: To build the aerobic base, neuromuscular speed and swimming efficiency

What: Warm up 5-10 minutes.

Swim 20-40 minutes continuously, repeating the following pattern for the duration of the swim: 25 easy free, 25 moderate free, 25 fast free, 25 easy backstroke.

Warm down.

Where: Pool

How: Use perceived exertion to monitor intensity

Swim (Fartlek 25s & Drills)

When: All training phases, especially base training

Why: To build the aerobic base, neuromuscular speed and swimming efficiency

What: Warm up: 500 easy

20 x 25 alternating between a fast "feel good speed" 25 (i.e. go as fast as you can without breaking form) and an easy 25 any stroke. You can go as slow as you need on the easy 25s, but aim to keep moving throughout the set.

*If you are in a 50-meter pool, note the halfway point for your 25s.

For the rest of your workout, do some easy swimming and drills that target areas you need to improve.

Warm down: 100 easy

Where: Pool

How: Use perceived exertion to monitor intensity

Swim (Fartlek in Open Water)

When: All training phases, especially base training

Why: To build the aerobic base, neuromuscular speed and swimming efficiency

What: Warm up 5-10 minutes.

Swim 20-40 minutes continuously, repeating the following pattern for the duration of the swim: 45 seconds easy free, 30 seconds moderate free, 15 seconds fast free, 30 seconds easy backstroke. Times are approximate; go by feel rather than worrying about exact times.

Warm down.

Where: Open water

How: Use perceived exertion to monitor intensity

Swim (Endurance with Build 25s)

When: All training phases, especially base training

Why: To condition fast-twitch and intermediate fast-twitch muscle fibers, and to develop the body's supporting structures (e.g. muscles, ligaments, tendons) that need to be in place for higher intensity aerobic and anaerobic work down the road

What: Warm up: 400 free, 200 backstroke, 200 rotating kick.

Swim 2 x 500 free in Zones 1-2 or at "easy" to "conversational" pace with 30 seconds rest.

Swim 10-20 x 25 free that build to maximum effort sprint with rest interval equal to work interval (set a send-off time based on swimming pace). Use fins if desired.

200 backstroke at recovery pace.

Optional: 200-500 pull in Zones 1-2 or at "easy" to "conversational" pace. Focus on body roll and breathing to alternate sides.

Warm down: 200 easy backstroke.

Where: Pool (long course)

How: Use perceived exertion and pace to monitor intensity

Swim (Aerobic Base 100s)

When: All training phases, especially base training

Why: To build the aerobic base by developing the ability to better metabolize fat and spare glycogen (stored carbohydrate) as a long duration energy source

What: Warm up: 400 free, 200 non-free and/or kick, 200 drill.

Swim 10-20 x 100 free in Zone 2 or at "conversational" pace with 15 seconds rest interval (set a send-off time based on your swimming pace zones). Focus on a steady pace.

Warm down: 200 easy backstroke.

Note: Choose number of 100s based on your send-off time so that you can finish the set in about 30 minutes. For example, if you swim the 100s in 1:15 your send-off time would be 1:30; this would allow you to do 20 x 100s in 30 minutes. Or, if you swim the 100s in 1:45 your send-off time would be 2:00; this would allow you to do 15 x 100s in 30 minutes. The entire workout should take about an hour, including warmup, main set, and warmdown.

Where: Pool

How: Use pace to monitor intensity

Swim (Aerobic Base 200s with Alactic 25s)

When: All training phases, especially base training

Why: To build the aerobic base, neuromuscular speed and swimming efficiency

What: Warm up: 400 free, 300 pull, 200 backstroke, 100 kick.

Swim 16 x 25 build freestyle (i.e. build to a sprint) with rest interval equivalent to swim time. Focus on good push off wall with nice streamline. Build to full speed and hold it for up to 10 seconds. This should be "feel good" speed.

Swim 8-10 x 200 free in Zone 2 or at "conversational" pace with 25 seconds rest interval (set a send-off time based on swimming pace zones). Focus on a steady pace.

Optional: 3-500 pull in Zone 2 or at "conversational" pace with backstroke every fourth 25. Focus on body roll and breathing to alternate sides. If you feel comfortable breathing every three strokes; then try to extend it to every five strokes.

Swim 8 x 50 with hands closed in fist during the first 25 of each 50. Focus on keeping the elbow high and finding the most effective position for your arm during the pull phase of your stroke. Open up fist and swim normally for second 25 of each 50. Focus on keeping elbow high and building upon the position you found during the fists drill. 15 seconds rest interval. Focus is on form not speed.

Warm down: 200 easy backstroke.

Where: Pool

How: Use pace or perceived exertion to monitor intensity

Swim (Aerobic Base 300s with Alactic 25s)

When: All training phases, especially base training

Why: To build the aerobic base, neuromuscular speed and swimming efficiency

What: Warm up: 400 free, 300 pull, 200 backstroke, 100 kick.

Swim 16 x 25 build freestyle (i.e. build to a sprint) with rest interval equivalent to swim time. Focus on good push off wall with nice streamline. Build to full speed and hold it for up to 10 seconds. This should be "feel good" speed.

Swim 6-8 x 300 free in Zone 2 or at "conversational" pace with 25 seconds rest interval (set a send-off time based on swimming pace zones). Focus on a steady pace.

Optional: 3-500 pull in Zone 2 or at "conversational" pace with backstroke every fourth 25. Focus on body roll and breathing to alternate sides. If you feel comfortable breathing every three strokes; then try to extend it to every five strokes.

Swim 8 x 50 with hands closed in fist during the first 25 of each 50. Focus on keeping the elbow high and finding the most effective position for your arm during the pull phase of your stroke. Open up fist and swim normally for second 25 of each 50. Focus on keeping elbow high and building upon the position you found during the fists drill. 15 seconds rest interval. Focus is on form not speed.

Warm down: 200 easy backstroke.

Where: Pool

How: Use pace or perceived exertion to monitor intensity

Swim (Aerobic Base 400s with Alactic 25s)

When: All training phases, especially base training

Why: To build the aerobic base, neuromuscular speed and swimming efficiency

What: Warm up: 400 free, 300 pull, 200 backstroke, 100 kick.

Swim 20 x 25 build freestyle (i.e. build to a sprint) with rest interval equivalent to swim time. Focus on good push off wall with nice streamline. Build to full speed and hold it for up to 10 seconds. This should be "feel good" speed.
Swim 200 backstroke for recovery.

Swim 4-6 x 400 free in Zone 2 or at "conversational" pace with 40 seconds rest interval (set a send-off time based on swimming pace zones). Focus on a steady pace.

Optional: 3-500 pull in Zone 2 or at "conversational" pace with backstroke every fourth 25. Focus on body roll and breathing to alternate sides. If you feel comfortable breathing every three strokes; then try to extend it to every five strokes.

Swim 6 x 50 drill for first 25 and build freestyle for last 25. 20 seconds rest interval. Focus on form.

Warm down: 200 easy backstroke.

Where: Pool

How: Use pace or perceived exertion to monitor intensity

Swim (Aerobic Base 500s with Alactic 25s)

When: All training phases, especially base training

Why: To build the aerobic base, neuromuscular speed and swimming efficiency

What: Warm up: 400 free, 300 pull, 200 backstroke, 100 kick.

Swim 20 x 25 build freestyle (i.e. build to a sprint) with rest interval equivalent to swim time. Focus on good push off wall with nice streamline. Build to full speed and hold it for up to 10 seconds. This should be "feel good" speed.

Swim 200 backstroke for recovery.

Swim 4-6 x 500 free in Zone 2 or at "conversational" pace with 50 seconds rest interval (set a send-off time based on swimming pace zones). Focus on a steady pace.

Swim 6 x 50 drill for first 25 and build freestyle for last 25. 20 seconds rest interval. Focus on form.

Warm down: 200 easy backstroke.

Where: Pool

How: Use pace or perceived exertion to monitor intensity

Swim (Aerobic Base 600s with Alactic 25s)

When: All training phases, especially base training

Why: To build the aerobic base, neuromuscular speed and swimming efficiency

What: Warm up: 400 free, 300 pull, 200 backstroke, 100 kick.

Swim 16 x 25 build freestyle (i.e. build to a sprint) with rest interval equivalent to swim time. Focus on good push off wall with nice streamline. Build to full speed and hold it for up to 10 seconds. This should be "feel good" speed.

Swim 200 backstroke for recovery.

Swim 4-6 x 600 free in Zone 2 or at "conversational" pace with 50 seconds rest interval (set a send-off time based on swimming pace zones). Focus on a steady pace.

Swim 6 x 50 drill for first 25 and recovery backstroke for last 25. 15 seconds rest interval. Focus on form.

Warm down: 200 easy backstroke.

Where: Pool

How: Use pace or perceived exertion to monitor intensity

Swim (Aerobic Base 800s)

When: All training phases, especially base training

Why: To build the aerobic base by developing the ability to better metabolize fat and spare glycogen (stored carbohydrate) as a long duration energy source

What: Warm up: 400 free, 300 pull, 200 backstroke, 100 kick.

Swim 3-5 x 800 free in Zone 2 or at "conversational" pace with 60 seconds rest interval. Focus on a steady pace.

Warm down: 200 easy backstroke.

Where: Pool

How: Use pace or perceived exertion to monitor intensity

Swim (Aerobic Base 1000s)

When: All training phases, especially base training

Why: To build the aerobic base by developing the ability to better metabolize fat and spare glycogen (stored carbohydrate) as a long duration energy source

What: Warm up: 400 free, 300 pull, 200 backstroke, 100 kick.

Swim 3-4 x 1,000 free in Zone 2 or at "conversational" pace with 60 seconds rest interval. Focus on a steady pace.

Warm down: 200 easy backstroke.

Where: Pool

How: Use pace or perceived exertion to monitor intensity

Aerobic Tempo Workouts

Swim (Base Tempo 75s)

When: Base training

Why: To build the aerobic base and improve lactate tolerance

What: Warm up: 400 free, 200 backstroke, 200 rotating kick.

Swim 6-12 x 75 free in Zone 3 or at "comfortably hard" pace with 10 seconds rest interval (set a send-off time based on swimming pace zones).

300 pull in Zones 1-2 or at "easy" to "conversational" pace. Focus on body roll and breathing to alternate sides.

Swim 6-12 x 75 in Zone 3 or at "comfortably hard" pace with 10 seconds rest interval (set a send-off time based on swimming pace zones).

6 x 50 with rotating kick for first 25 and build freestyle for second 25. Take a 20 second rest interval.

Warm down: 200 easy backstroke.

Where: Pool

How: Use pace or perceived exertion to monitor intensity

Swim (Base Tempo 100s)

When: Base training

Why: To build the aerobic base and improve lactate tolerance

What: Warm up: 400 free, 200 backstroke, 200 rotating kick.

Swim 8-10 x 100 free in Zone 3 or at "comfortably hard" pace with 20 seconds rest interval (set a send-off time based on swimming pace zones).

200 backstroke in Zone 1 or at "easy" pace.

Swim 8-10 x 100 free in Zone 3 or at "comfortably hard" pace with 20 seconds rest interval (set a send-off time based on swimming pace zones).

6 x 50 with rotating kick for first 25 and build freestyle for second 25 with 20 seconds rest interval.
Warm down: 200 easy backstroke.

Where: Pool

How: Use pace or perceived exertion to monitor intensity

Swim (Base Tempo 200s)

When: Base training

Why: To build the aerobic base and improve lactate tolerance

What: Warm up: 400 free, 200 backstroke, 200 rotating kick.

Swim 4-5 x 200 free in Zone 3 or at "comfortably hard" pace with 25 seconds rest interval (set a send-off time based on swimming pace zones).

200 backstroke in Zone 1 or at "easy" pace.

Swim 4-5 x 200 free in Zone 3 or at "comfortably hard" pace with 25 seconds rest interval (set a send-off time based on swimming pace zones).

6 x 50 with rotating kick for first 25 and non-free recovery swim for second 25. 15 seconds rest interval.

Warm down: 200 easy backstroke.

Where: Pool

How: Use pace or perceived exertion to monitor intensity

Swim (Base Tempo 300s)

When: Base training

Why: To build the aerobic base and improve lactate tolerance

What: Warm up: 400 free, 200 backstroke, 200 rotating kick.

Swim 3-4 x 300 free in Zone 3 or at "comfortably hard" pace with 30 seconds rest interval (set a send-off time based on swimming pace zones).
200 backstroke in Zone 1 or at "easy" pace.

Swim 3-4 x 300 free in Zone 3 or at "comfortably hard" pace with 30 seconds rest interval (set a send-off time based on swimming pace zones).

6 x 50 with rotating kick for first 25 and recovery backstroke for second 25 with 15 seconds rest interval.

Warm down: 200 easy backstroke.

Where: Pool

How: Use pace or perceived exertion to monitor intensity

Swim (Base Tempo 400s)

When: Base training

Why: To build the aerobic base and improve lactate tolerance

What: Warm up: 400 free, 200 backstroke, 200 rotating kick.

Swim 2-3 x 400 free in Zone 3 or at "comfortably hard" pace with 40 seconds rest interval (set a send-off time based on swimming pace zones).

200 backstroke in Zone 1 or at "easy" pace.

Swim 2-3 x 400 free in Zone 3 or at "comfortably hard" pace with 40 seconds rest interval (set a send-off time based on swimming pace zones).

12 x 25 free sprints. Rest interval is equivalent to swim time.

Warm down: 200 easy backstroke.

Where: Pool

How: Use pace or perceived exertion to monitor intensity

Swim (Base Tempo 500s)

When: Base training

Why: To build the aerobic base and improve lactate tolerance

What: Warm up: 400 free, 200 backstroke, 200 rotating kick.

Swim 3-4 x 500 free in Zone 3 or at "comfortably hard" pace with 50 seconds rest interval.

200 backstroke in Zone 1 or at "easy" pace.

4-12 x 25 free sprints with rest interval equivalent to swim time.

Warm down: 200 easy backstroke.

Where: Pool

How: Use pace or perceived exertion to monitor intensity

Threshold Workouts

Swim (LT Cruise 300s)

When: Late base training; build training; peak training

Why: To raise the lactate threshold by improving lactate tolerance and decreasing lactate accumulation (which allows you to stay aerobic as faster speeds)

What: Warm up: 400 free, 200 backstroke, 200 rotating kick.

Swim 1-2 x 300 free in Zones 4-5a or at "comfortably hard" pace with 30 seconds rest interval (set a send-off time based on swimming pace zones).

200 backstroke at "easy" pace.

Swim 1-2 x 300 free in Zones 4-5a or at "comfortably hard" pace with 30 seconds rest interval (set a send-off time based on swimming pace zones).

200 backstroke at "easy" pace.

Optional: 200-500 pull in Zones 1-2 or at "easy" to "conversational" pace. Focus on body roll and breathing to alternate sides.

Warm down: 200 easy backstroke.

Where: Pool

How: Use pace or perceived exertion to monitor intensity

Swim (LT Cruise 400s)

When: Late base training; build training; peak training

Why: To raise the lactate threshold by improving lactate tolerance and decreasing lactate accumulation (which allows you to stay aerobic as faster speeds)

What: Warm up: 400 free, 200 backstroke, 200 rotating kick.

Swim 2-3 x 400 free in Zones 4-5a or at "comfortably hard" pace with 40 seconds rest interval (set a send-off time based on swimming pace zones).

200 backstroke in Zone 1 or at "easy" pace.

Optional: 200-500 pull in Zones 1-2 or at "easy" to

"conversational" pace. Focus on body roll and breathing to alternate sides.

Warm down: 200 easy backstroke.

Where: Pool

How: Use pace or perceived exertion to monitor intensity

Swim (LT Cruise 500s)

When: Late base training; build training; peak training

Why: To raise the lactate threshold by improving lactate tolerance and decreasing lactate accumulation (which allows you to stay aerobic as faster speeds)

What: Warm up: 400 free, 200 backstroke, 200 rotating kick.

Swim 1-3 x 500 free in Zones 4-5a or at "comfortably hard" pace with 50 seconds rest interval (set a send-off time based on swimming pace zones).

200 backstroke in Zone 1 or at "easy" pace.

Optional: 200-500 pull in Zones 1-2 or at "easy" to "conversational" pace. Focus on body roll and breathing to alternate sides.

Warm down: 200 easy backstroke.

Where: Pool

How: Use pace or perceived exertion to monitor intensity

V_{O_2} Max Workouts

Swim (VO_2 200s)

When: Build training; peak training

Why: To increase the maximal rate of oxygen transport (aerobic capacity or VO2max), build lactate tolerance, and increase anaerobic endurance

What: Warm up: 400 free, 200 backstroke, 200 rotating kick.

Swim 2-3 x 200 free in Zone 5b or at "uncomfortably hard" pace with 50 easy swim plus 15 seconds rest interval (set a send-off time based on swimming pace zones).
200 backstroke in Zone 1 or at "easy" pace.

Swim 2-3 x 200 free in Zone 5b or at "uncomfortably hard" pace with 50 easy swim plus 15 seconds rest interval (set a send-off time based on swimming pace zones).

200 backstroke in Zone 1 or at "easy" pace.

Optional: 200-500 pull in Zones 1-2 or at "easy" to "conversational" pace. Focus on body roll and breathing to alternate sides.

Warm down: 200 easy backstroke.

Where: Pool

How: Use pace or perceived exertion to monitor intensity

Swim (VO₂ 300s)

When: Build training; peak training

Why: To increase the maximal rate of oxygen transport (aerobic capacity or VO2max), build lactate tolerance, and increase anaerobic endurance

What: Warm up: 400 free, 200 backstroke, 200 rotating kick.

Swim 1-2 x 300 free in Zone 5b or at "uncomfortably hard" pace with 50 easy swim plus 30 seconds rest interval (set a send-off time based on swimming pace zones).

200 backstroke in Zone 1 or at "easy" pace.

Swim 1-2 x 300 free in Zone 5b or at "uncomfortably hard" pace with 50 easy swim plus 30 seconds rest interval (set a send-off time based on swimming pace zones).

200 backstroke in Zone 1 or at "easy" pace.

Optional: 200-500 pull in Zones 1-2 or at "easy" to "conversational" pace. Focus on body roll and breathing to alternate sides.

Warm down: 200 easy backstroke.

Where: Pool

How: Use pace or perceived exertion to monitor intensity

Anaerobic Capacity Workouts

Swim (Speed Rep 50s)

When: Build training; peak training

Why: To improve the ability to maintain short durations of speed of up to 2 minutes in duration (starts, race surges, finishing kicks)

What: Warm up: 400 free, 200 backstroke, 200 rotating kick.

Swim 8-16 x 50 free in Zone 5c or at "all out" pace with rest interval equal to work interval (set a send-off time based on swimming pace).

200 backstroke in Zone 1 or at "easy" pace.

Optional: 200-500 pull in Zones 1-2 or at "easy" to "conversational" pace. Focus on body roll and breathing to alternate sides.

Warm down: 200 easy backstroke.

Where: Pool

How: Use pace or perceived exertion to monitor intensity

Swim (Speed Rep 75s)

When: Build training; peak training

Why: To improve the ability to maintain short durations of speed of up to 2 minutes in duration (starts, race surges, finishing kicks)

What: Warm up: 400 free, 200 backstroke, 200 rotating kick.

Swim 3-6 x 75 free in Zone 5c or at "all out" pace with 25 easy swim plus 60 seconds rest interval in between (set a send-off time based on swimming pace).

200 backstroke in Zone 1 or at "easy" pace.

Swim 3-6 x 75 free in Zone 5c or at "all out" pace with 25 easy swim plus 60 seconds rest interval in between (set a send-off time based on swimming pace).

200 backstroke in Zone 1 or at "easy" pace.

Optional: 200-500 pull in Zones 1-2 or at "easy" to "conversational" pace. Focus on body roll and breathing to alternate sides.

Warm down: 200 easy backstroke.

Where: Pool

How: Use pace or perceived exertion to monitor intensity

Swim (Speed Rep 100s)

When: Build training; peak training

Why: To improve the ability to maintain short durations of speed of up to 2 minutes in duration (starts, race surges, finishing kicks)

What: Warm up: 400 free, 200 backstroke, 200 rotating kick.

Swim 2-4 x 100 free in Zone 5c or at "all out" pace with rest interval equal to work interval (set a send-off time based on swimming pace).

200 backstroke in Zone 1 or at "easy" pace.

Swim 2-4 x 100 free in Zone 5c or at "all out" pace with rest interval equal to work interval (set a send-off time based on swimming pace).

200 backstroke in Zone 1 or at "easy" pace.

Optional: 200-500 pull in Zones 1-2 or at "easy" to "conversational" pace. Focus on body roll and breathing to alternate sides.

Warm down: 200 easy backstroke.

Where: Pool

How: Use pace or perceived exertion to monitor intensity

Swimming Drills

Catch-up Drill

Have you ever noticed how the faster boats are the longer boats (think a rowing team's racing shell versus a fisherman's rowboat)?

The same physics that apply to building a fast racing boat apply to the human body moving through the water. The catch-up drill will help you focus on maintaining a long body in the water.

To do the drill, maintain your non-stroking arm in front of you in its initial extended position. Then wait until the stroking arm "catches up" with your extended arm before taking your next stroke.

This effectively slows down your swimming, and allows you to focus on stroking with one arm at a time. But more importantly, it shifts your center of gravity forward a bit to give you a more balanced body position. In addition, it gives you a longer profile more like a racing shell than a barge.

For swimmers who have a tendency to rush through the initial extension phase, aim for a ¾ catch-up while swimming at your aerobic base pace to ingrain this longer body position into your new habits.

Single Arm Drill (Variation 1)

This drill isolates one arm at a time to focus on your stroke.

Keep the non-stroking arm extended in front of the body (held in the extended post-entry phase).

As you enter with the stroking arm, focus on keeping the elbow high and rolling to that side to work on proper body roll.

Exhale as you stroke, completing your exhalation before the stroking arm leaves the water.

Breathe to the side of your working arm.

Single Arm Drill (Variation 2)

In this variation of the single arm drill, keep your non-stroking arm down at your side. (In other words, the hand of the non-stroking arm is at the hip.)

As you enter with the stroking arm, focus on keeping the elbow high and rolling to that side to work on proper body roll.

Breathe to the side of the non-working arm.

Fists Drill

Instead of swimming with paddles, the fists drill is more like swimming with anti-paddles. Just as the name implies, close up your hands into fists and swim.

If you feel like you aren't getting very far, remember to keep your elbow high during the pull phase of the stroke. Let your arm seek out the optimal position that grips the water and provides the most power.

If you have a tendency to drop your elbow and let your arm slip through the water, this drill will provide the feedback you need to develop a better 'feel' for proper arm positioning during your stroke.

Finger-tip Drag Drill

This drill allows you to work on the recovery portion of the stroke.

As you lift your arm out of the water for the recovery, imagine a string tied to your elbow. Keep your arm relaxed and let this imaginary string lift your arm by your elbow and carry it around to the entry of your next stroke. This is the basic idea of how the bent-arm recovery should feel.

The finger-tip drag drill provides you with more kinesthetic feedback. To do the drill, let your fingertips skim across the surface of the water during the recovery phase. This will help you gain a better feel for the correct positioning of the bent-arm during recovery.

Thumb to Thigh Brush Drill

The last third of the stroke generates the most power and propulsion. Thus, a good follow-through is crucial to a powerful stroke. This drill helps reinforce full extension of your arm at the end of the stroke.

Simply brush your thumb against the side of your thigh as you finish; this will give you a target for where your hand should be finishing—namely, by your thigh with arm extended (rather than pulling out earlier by your hip).

Rotating, or Side-to-Side Kick

Freestyle and backstroke are both "side to side" strokes in that the swimmer rotates along the spine of the body. This kick also doubles as a type of drill insofar as it develops body roll along this axis.

The kick is done without a board; fins are encouraged. Start off lying on one side with your bottom arm extended above your head and your top arm at your side. Kick about six times; then take a stroke and rotate to the other side. Repeat.

With this kick, you are effectively freezing your stroke—bottom arm in extended entry position, top arm in extended follow-through position—while you kick. As you take a stroke to rotate to the other side, focus on gradually accelerating from the beginning to end of that stroke. Finish with a nice snap of the hips as you roll the body.

When you are comfortable with the basic rotating kick; then add a sculling motion with your bottom arm (i.e. the arm extended in the entry position). Scull by medially and laterally rotating the forearm. Sculpt the water with your hand. After six kicks, move from the sculling motion into your stroke to roll onto the other side.

Fashion Model Backstroke Kick

An effective body roll can also be achieved by practicing backstroke. For this drill, you are kicking on your back with both arms down at your side. Use fins if you have them. While kicking, move one shoulder to your chin, allowing your body to roll to the side. Then do the same to the other side, rotating from side to side along your spinal axis.

10
BIKE WORKOUTS

Recovery Workouts

Bike (Easy)

When: Any training phase

Why: To aid recovery, add to your training volume and loosen you up for the key workouts of the week

What: Bike primarily in Zones 1-2 or at "easy" to "conversational" pace. Keep cadence high (90 rpm or above). Don't worry about pace; goal is to loosen legs and feel fresh at end.

Where: Flats or trainer

How: Use heart rate or perceived exertion to monitor intensity

Bike (Easy with Isolated Leg Drill)

When: Any training phase

Why: To aid recovery, add to your training volume, work on form

What: Bike primarily in Zones 1-2 or at "easy" to "conversational" pace. Keep cadence high (90 rpm or above). Don't worry about pace; goal is to loosen legs and feel fresh at end. After you are warmed up, perform several repetitions of the isolated leg drill. This drill is best done on a stationary trainer or a flat road with not traffic or distractions. Unclip one leg from the pedals, and spin in circles with the other leg. Focus on smooth pedal stroke with a cadence of 90 rpm or above. Do this for 10-30 seconds per leg; then switch legs. Pedal normally in between repetitions.

Where: Flats or trainer

How: Use heart rate or perceived exertion to monitor intensity

Bike (Easy with Spin-ups)

When: Any training phase

Why: To aid recovery, add to your training volume, work on form

What: Bike primarily in Zones 1-2 or at "easy" to "conversational" pace. Keep cadence high (90 rpm or above). Don't worry about pace; goal is to loosen legs and feel fresh at end. After you are warmed up, perform several "spin-ups" by gradually increasing your cadence as high as possible (without bouncing) and hold for as long as possible (up to a minute). Recover for at least a minute before repeating. Don't worry about heart rate during the spin-ups.

Where: Flats or trainer

How: Use heart rate or perceived exertion to monitor intensity

Bike (Easy with Short Sprints)

When: Any training phase

Why: To aid recovery, add to your training volume and develop neuromuscular speed

What: Bike primarily in Zones 1-2 or at "easy" to "conversational" pace. Keep cadence high (90 rpm or above). During the ride, find a flat straightaway. Once you are warmed up, perform 4-12 x accelerations where you build to a maximum effort sprint and hold that sprint for up to 10 seconds. Ride at an "easy" pace for about 3-5 minutes in between each sprint.

Where: Flats or trainer

How: Use heart rate or perceived exertion to monitor intensity

Bike (Pre-race Warmup)

When: Day before a race

Why: To loosen up, check equipment, and scout out the course

What: This is effectively an "active rest day." Your aim is get in a short warm up to check equipment and loosen up.

You will have a lot of energy, especially with the excitement of race week. But remember that today is not the race nor is it a day for an extended workout. Do just enough to get the blood flowing, keeping it in Zone 1 with a few spin-ups or short sprints.

Stay hydrated and fueled. Eat well, and relax in preparation for the race.

Where: Race course (if possible) or stationary trainer

How: Use perceived exertion and pace to monitor intensity

Endurance Workouts

Bike (Endurance Ride)

When: All training phases, especially base training

Why: To build the aerobic base by developing the ability to better metabolize fat and spare glycogen (stored carbohydrate) as a long duration energy source

What: Bike primarily in Zone 2 or at "conversational" pace. Keep cadence at 90 rpm or above.

Where: Flats, hills, trainer

How: Use heart rate or perceived exertion to monitor intensity

Bike (Endurance Ride with Spin-ups)

When: All training phases, especially base training

Why: To build the aerobic base and neuromuscular speed

What: Bike primarily in Zone 2 or at "conversational" pace. Keep cadence at 90 rpm or above. After you are warmed up, perform several "spin-ups" by gradually increasing your cadence as high as possible (without bouncing) and hold for as long as possible (up to a minute). Recover for at least a minute before repeating. Don't worry about heart rate during the spin-ups.

Where: Flats, hills, trainer

How: Use heart rate or perceived exertion to monitor intensity

Bike (Endurance Ride with Short Sprints)

When: All training phases, especially base training

Why: To build the aerobic base and neuromuscular speed

What: Bike primarily in Zone 2 or at "conversational" pace. Keep cadence at 90 rpm or above. During the ride, find a flat straightaway. Once you are warmed up, perform 4-12 x accelerations where you build to a maximum effort sprint and hold that sprint for up to 10 seconds. Ride at an "easy" pace for about 3-5 minutes in between each sprint.

Where: Flats, trainer

How: Use heart rate or perceived exertion to monitor intensity

Bike (Endurance Ride with Short Hills)

When: All training phases, especially base training

Why: To build the aerobic base, neuromuscular speed and power

What: Bike primarily in Zone 2 or at "conversational" pace. Keep cadence at 90 rpm or above. During the ride, find a hill with a grade of about 4-8 percent. Once you are warmed up, perform 4-12 x accelerations where you build to a maximum effort sprint and hold that sprint for up to 10 seconds. Ride at an "easy" pace for about 3-5 minutes in between each hill repeat.

Where: Hills

How: Use heart rate or perceived exertion to monitor intensity

Bike (Long Ride)

When: All training phases, especially base training

Why: To build the aerobic base by developing the ability to better metabolize fat and spare glycogen (stored carbohydrate) as a long duration energy source

What: Bike primarily in Zone 2 or at "conversational" pace. Keep cadence at 90 rpm or above.

Where: Flats, hills, trainer

How: Use heart rate or perceived exertion to monitor intensity

Aerobic Tempo Workouts

Bike (20-min Base Tempo)

When: Base training

Why: To build the aerobic base and improve lactate tolerance

What: Once you are thoroughly warmed up (at least 15-20 minutes), up your tempo into Zone 3 or at "comfortably hard" pace for 20 minutes. When finished with the tempo, do the remainder of the ride in Zones 1-2 or at "easy" to "conversational" pace. As always, focus on keeping your cadence at 90 or above throughout the ride.

Where: Flats, hills, trainer

How: Use heart rate or perceived exertion to monitor intensity

Bike (30-min Base Tempo)

When: Base training

Why: To build the aerobic base and improve lactate tolerance

What: Once you are thoroughly warmed up (at least 15-20 minutes), up your tempo into Zone 3 or at "comfortably hard" pace for 30 minutes. When finished with the tempo, do the remainder of the ride in Zones 1-2 or at "easy" to "conversational" pace. As always, focus on keeping your cadence at 90 or above throughout the ride.

Where: Flats, hills, trainer

How: Use heart rate or perceived exertion to monitor intensity

Bike (40-min Base Tempo)

When: Base training

Why: To build the aerobic base and improve lactate tolerance

What: Once you are thoroughly warmed up (at least 15-20 minutes), up your tempo into Zone 3 or at "comfortably hard" pace for 40 minutes. When finished with the tempo, do the remainder of the ride in Zones 1-2 or at "easy" to "conversational" pace. As always, focus on keeping your cadence at 90 or above throughout the ride.

Where: Flats, hills, trainer

How: Use heart rate or perceived exertion to monitor intensity

Threshold Workouts

Bike (Sub-LT Cruise Intervals 5/1)

When: Late base training; build training; peak training

Why: To raise the lactate threshold by improving lactate tolerance and decreasing lactate accumulation (which allows you to

stay aerobic as faster speeds)

What: Once you are thoroughly warmed up (at least 15-20 minutes), perform up to 12 x 5-min work interval in Zone 4 or at "comfortably hard" pace followed by 1-min recovery interval. When finished with the intervals, do the remainder of ride in Zones 1-2 or at "easy" to "conversational" pace ensuring that you complete an adequate warm down (at least 10 minutes). As always, focus on keeping your cadence at 90 or above throughout the ride, including the recovery intervals.

Where: Flats, hills, trainer

How: Use heart rate or perceived exertion to monitor intensity

Bike (Sub-LT Cruise Intervals 8/2)

When: Late base training; build training; peak training

Why: To raise the lactate threshold by improving lactate tolerance and decreasing lactate accumulation (which allows you to stay aerobic as faster speeds)

What: Once you are thoroughly warmed up (at least 15-20 minutes), perform up to 7 x 8-min work interval in Zone 4 or at "comfortably hard" pace followed by 2-min recovery interval. When finished with the intervals, do the remainder of ride in Zones 1-2 or at "easy" to "conversational" pace ensuring that you complete an adequate warm down (at least 10 minutes). As always, focus on keeping your cadence at 90 or above throughout the ride, including the recovery intervals.

Where: Flats, hills, trainer

How: Use heart rate or perceived exertion to monitor intensity

Bike (Sub-LT Cruise Intervals 10/2)

When: Late base training; build training; peak training

Why: To raise the lactate threshold by improving lactate tolerance and decreasing lactate accumulation (which allows you to

stay aerobic as faster speeds)

What: Once you are thoroughly warmed up (at least 15-20 minutes), perform up to 6 x 10-min work interval in Zone 4 or at "comfortably hard" pace followed by 2-min recovery interval. When finished with the intervals, do the remainder of ride in Zones 1-2 or at "easy" to "conversational" pace ensuring that you complete an adequate warm down (at least 10 minutes). As always, focus on keeping your cadence at 90 or above throughout the ride, including the recovery intervals.

Where: Flats, hills, trainer

How: Use heart rate or perceived exertion to monitor intensity

Bike (Sub-LT 20-minute Tempo)

When: Late base training; build training; peak training

Why: To raise the lactate threshold by improving lactate tolerance and decreasing lactate accumulation (which allows you to stay aerobic as faster speeds)

What: Once you are thoroughly warmed up (at least 15-20 minutes), up your tempo into Zone 4 or "comfortably hard" pace for 20 minutes. When finished with the tempo interval, do the remainder of the ride in Zones 1-2 or at "easy" to "conversational" pace. As always, focus on keeping your cadence at 90 or above throughout the ride.

Where: Flats, hills, trainer

How: Use heart rate or perceived exertion to monitor intensity

Bike (Sub-LT 30-minute Tempo)

When: Late base training; build training; peak training

Why: To raise the lactate threshold by improving lactate tolerance and decreasing lactate accumulation (which allows you to stay aerobic as faster speeds)

What: Once you are thoroughly warmed up (at least 15-20

minutes), up your tempo into Zone 4 or "comfortably hard" pace for 30 minutes. When finished with the tempo interval, do the remainder of the ride in Zones 1-2 or at "easy" to "conversational" pace. As always, focus on keeping your cadence at 90 or above throughout the ride.

Where: Flats, hills, trainer

How: Use heart rate or perceived exertion to monitor intensity

Bike (Sub-LT 40-minute Tempo)

When: Late base training; build training; peak training

Why: To raise the lactate threshold by improving lactate tolerance and decreasing lactate accumulation (which allows you to stay aerobic as faster speeds)

What: Once you are thoroughly warmed up (at least 15-20 minutes), up your tempo into Zone 4 or "comfortably hard" pace for 40 minutes. When finished with the tempo interval, do the remainder of the ride in Zones 1-2 or at "easy" to "conversational" pace. As always, focus on keeping your cadence at 90 or above throughout the ride.

Where: Flats, hills, trainer

How: Use heart rate or perceived exertion to monitor intensity

Bike (Sub-LT 60-minute Tempo)

When: Late base training; build training; peak training

Why: To raise the lactate threshold by improving lactate tolerance and decreasing lactate accumulation (which allows you to stay aerobic as faster speeds)

What: Once you are thoroughly warmed up (at least 15-20 minutes), up your tempo into Zone 4 or "comfortably hard" pace for 60 minutes. When finished with the tempo interval, do the remainder of the ride in Zones 1-2 or at "easy" to "conversational" pace. As always, focus on keeping your cadence at 90 or above throughout the ride.

Where: Flats, hills, trainer

How: Use heart rate or perceived exertion to monitor intensity

Bike (LT Cruise Intervals 5/1)

When: Late base training; build training; peak training

Why: To raise the lactate threshold by improving lactate tolerance and decreasing lactate accumulation (which allows you to stay aerobic as faster speeds)

What: Once you are thoroughly warmed up (at least 15-20 minutes), perform up to 12 x 5-min work interval in Zones 4-5a or at "comfortably hard" pace followed by 1-min recovery interval. When finished with the intervals, do the remainder of ride in Zones 1-2 or at "easy" to "conversational" pace ensuring that you complete an adequate warm down (at least 10 minutes). As always, focus on keeping your cadence at 90 or above throughout the ride, including the recovery intervals.

Where: Flats, hills, trainer

How: Use heart rate or perceived exertion to monitor intensity

Bike (LT Cruise Intervals 8/2)

When: Late base training; build training; peak training

Why: To raise the lactate threshold by improving lactate tolerance and decreasing lactate accumulation (which allows you to stay aerobic as faster speeds)

What: Once you are thoroughly warmed up (at least 15-20 minutes), perform up to 7 x 8-min work interval in Zones 4-5a or at "comfortably hard" pace followed by 2-min recovery interval. When finished with the intervals, do the remainder of ride in Zones 1-2 or at "easy" to "conversational" pace ensuring that you complete an adequate warm down (at least 10 minutes). As always, focus on keeping your cadence at 90 or above throughout the ride, including the recovery intervals.

Where: Flats, hills, trainer

How: Use heart rate or perceived exertion to monitor intensity

Bike (LT Cruise Intervals 10/2)

When: Late base training; build training; peak training

Why: To raise the lactate threshold by improving lactate tolerance and decreasing lactate accumulation (which allows you to stay aerobic as faster speeds)

What: Once you are thoroughly warmed up (at least 15-20 minutes), perform up to 6 x 10-min work interval in Zones 4-5a or at "comfortably hard" pace followed by 2-min recovery interval. When finished with the intervals, do the remainder of ride in Zones 1-2 or at "easy" to "conversational" pace ensuring that you complete an adequate warm down (at least 10 minutes). As always, focus on keeping your cadence at 90 or above throughout the ride, including the recovery intervals.

Where: Flats, hills, trainer

How: Use heart rate or perceived exertion to monitor intensity

Bike (LT 20-minute Tempo)

When: Late base training; build training; peak training

Why: To raise the lactate threshold by improving lactate tolerance and decreasing lactate accumulation (which allows you to stay aerobic as faster speeds)

What: Once you are thoroughly warmed up (at least 15-20 minutes), up your tempo into Zones 4-5a or "comfortably hard" pace for 20 minutes. When finished with the tempo interval, do the remainder of the ride in Zones 1-2 or at "easy" to "conversational" pace. As always, focus on keeping your cadence at 90 or above throughout the ride.

Where: Flats, hills, trainer

How: Use heart rate or perceived exertion to monitor intensity

Bike (LT 30-minute Tempo)

When: Late base training; build training; peak training

Why: To raise the lactate threshold by improving lactate tolerance and decreasing lactate accumulation (which allows you to stay aerobic as faster speeds)

What: Once you are thoroughly warmed up (at least 15-20 minutes), up your tempo into Zones 4-5a or "comfortably hard" pace for 30 minutes. When finished with the tempo interval, do the remainder of the ride in Zones 1-2 or at "easy" to "conversational" pace. As always, focus on keeping your cadence at 90 or above throughout the ride.

Where: Flats, hills, trainer

How: Use heart rate or perceived exertion to monitor intensity

Bike (LT 40-minute Tempo)

When: Late base training; build training; peak training

Why: To raise the lactate threshold by improving lactate tolerance and decreasing lactate accumulation (which allows you to stay aerobic as faster speeds)

What: Once you are thoroughly warmed up (at least 15-20 minutes), up your tempo into Zones 4-5a or "comfortably hard" pace for 40 minutes. When finished with the tempo interval, do the remainder of the ride in Zones 1-2 or at "easy" to "conversational" pace. As always, focus on keeping your cadence at 90 or above throughout the ride.

Where: Flats, hills, trainer

How: Use heart rate or perceived exertion to monitor intensity

Bike (LT 60-minute Tempo)

When: Late base training; build training; peak training

Why: To raise the lactate threshold by improving lactate tolerance and decreasing lactate accumulation (which allows you to

stay aerobic as faster speeds)

What: Once you are thoroughly warmed up (at least 15-20 minutes), up your tempo into Zones 4-5a or "comfortably hard" pace for 60 minutes. When finished with the tempo interval, do the remainder of the ride in Zones 1-2 or at "easy" to "conversational" pace. As always, focus on keeping your cadence at 90 or above throughout the ride.

Where: Flats, hills, trainer

How: Use heart rate or perceived exertion to monitor intensity

VO_2 Max Workouts

Bike (VO_2 Intervals 3/2)

When: Build training; peak training

Why: To increase the maximal rate of oxygen transport (aerobic capacity or VO2max), build lactate tolerance, and increase anaerobic endurance

What: Once you are thoroughly warmed up (15-25 minutes), perform up to 9 x 3-min work interval in Zone 5b or "uncomfortably hard" pace followed by 2-min recovery interval. When finished with the intervals, do the remainder of the ride in Zones 1-2 or at "easy" to "conversational" pace ensuring that you complete an adequate warm down (at least 10 minutes). As always, focus on keeping your cadence at 90 or above throughout the ride, including the recovery intervals.

Where: Flats, hills, trainer

How: Use heart rate or perceived exertion to monitor intensity

Bike (VO_2 Intervals 4/3)

When: Build training; peak training

Why: To increase the maximal rate of oxygen transport (aerobic capacity or VO2max), build lactate tolerance, and increase anaerobic endurance

What: Once you are thoroughly warmed up (15-25 minutes), perform up to 7 x 4-min work interval in Zone 5b or "uncomfortably hard" pace followed by 3-min recovery interval. When finished with the intervals, do the remainder of the ride in Zones 1-2 or at "easy" to "conversational" pace ensuring that you complete an adequate warm down (at least 10 minutes). As always, focus on keeping your cadence at 90 or above throughout the ride, including the recovery intervals.

Where: Flats, hills, trainer

How: Use heart rate or perceived exertion to monitor intensity

Bike (VO$_2$ Intervals 5/4)

When: Build training; peak training

Why: To increase the maximal rate of oxygen transport (aerobic capacity or VO2max), build lactate tolerance, and increase anaerobic endurance

What: Once you are thoroughly warmed up (15-25 minutes), perform up to 6 x 5-min work interval in Zone 5b or "uncomfortably hard" pace followed by 4-min recovery interval. When finished with the intervals, do the remainder of the ride in Zones 1-2 or at "easy" to "conversational" pace ensuring that you complete an adequate warm down (at least 10 minutes). As always, focus on keeping your cadence at 90 or above throughout the ride, including the recovery intervals.

Where: Flats, hills, trainer

How: Use heart rate or perceived exertion to monitor intensity

Anaerobic Capacity Workouts

Bike (Speed Reps 1/2)

When: Build training; peak training

Why: To improve the ability to maintain short durations of speed of up to 2 minutes in duration (starts, race surges, kicks)

What: Once you are thoroughly warmed up (15-25 minutes), perform up to 10 x 1-min work interval in Zone 5c or "all out" pace followed by 2-min recovery interval. (Note: heart rate generally takes about 30 seconds to move into target zone so focus on being in Zone 5c over last part of the work interval.) When finished with the intervals, do the remainder of the ride at an easy pace (Zones 1-2) ensuring that you complete an adequate warm down (at least 10 minutes). As always, focus on keeping your cadence at 90 or above throughout the ride, including the recovery intervals.

Where: Flats, hills, trainer

How: Use heart rate or perceived exertion to monitor intensity

Bike (Speed Reps 2/4)

When: Build training; peak training

Why: To improve the ability to maintain short durations of speed of up to 2 minutes in duration (starts, race surges, finishing kicks)

What: Once you are thoroughly warmed up (15-25 minutes), perform up to 6 x 2-min work interval in Zone 5c or "all out" pace followed by 4-min recovery interval. (Note: heart rate generally takes about 30 seconds to move into target zone so focus on being in Zone 5c over last part of the work interval.) When finished with the intervals, do the remainder of the ride at an easy pace (Zones 1-2) ensuring that you complete an adequate warm down (at least 10 minutes). As always, focus on keeping your cadence at 90 or above throughout the ride, including the recovery intervals.

Where: Flats, hills, trainer

How: Use heart rate or perceived exertion to monitor intensity

11

RUN WORKOUTS

Recovery Workouts

Run (Easy)

When: Any training phase

Why: To aid recovery, add to your training volume and loosen you up for the key workouts of the week

What: Run primarily in Zones 1-2 or at "easy" to "conversational" pace. Focus on keeping cadence between at least 28-30 left foot strikes per 20 seconds (84-90 per minute). Don't worry about pace or distance covered; goal is to feel fresh at the end. This run is ideal to do on trails where you can keep it easy without worrying about time splits. Note: if you feel overly fatigued going into this workout, then cut back the duration of this run—or take the day off completely.

Where: Flats, hills, treadmill

How: Use heart rate, pace or perceived exertion to monitor intensity

Run (Easy with Short Acceleration Striders)

When: Any training phase

Why: To aid recovery, add to your training volume and develop neuromuscular speed

What: Run primarily in Zones 1-2 or at "easy" to "conversational" pace. Focus on keeping cadence between at least 28-30 left foot strikes per 20 seconds (84-90 per minute). Throughout the run, throw in 6-8 x short accelerations. Start off easy and gradually pick up your pace until you're at full speed. Hold full speed for up to 10 seconds; then wind it back down. These are "feel good" sprints—you want to feel good going fast. Focus on good form and leg turnover. Run easy for 2-3 minutes between each strider or until you feel fully recovered and ready for the next one. Don't worry about time or heart rate on the striders.

Where: Flats (grass, trail or track)

How: Use heart rate, pace or perceived exertion to monitor intensity

Run (Easy with Drill Session 1)

When: Any training phase

Why: To aid recovery, add to your training volume and work on form

What: This is an easy run with a focus on drills. Warm up for 10-20 minutes in Zone 1 or at "easy" pace; then spend about 10 minutes on the following drills before finishing the remainder of the run in Zones 1-2 or at "easy" to "conversational" pace.
- Loosening Skips
- Side Skips
- Straight Leg Run
- Butt Kicks

(see end of chapter for explanation of drills)

Where: Flats (grass, trail or track)

How: Use heart rate, pace or perceived exertion to monitor intensity

Run (Easy with Drill Session 2)

When: Any training phase

Why: To aid recovery, add to your training volume and work on form

What: This is an easy run with a focus on drills. Warm up for 10-20 minutes in Zone 1 or at "easy" pace; then spend about 10 minutes on the following drills before finishing the remainder of the run in Zones 1-2 or at "easy" to "conversational" pace.
- Loosening Skips
- Side Skips
- Carioca, or Grapevine
- Straight Leg Run
- Butt Kicks
- High Knees

(see end of chapter for explanation of drills)

Where: Flats (grass, trail or track)

How: Use heart rate, pace or perceived exertion to monitor intensity

Run (Easy with Drill Session 3)

When: Any training phase

Why: To aid recovery, add to your training volume and work on form

What: This is an easy run with a focus on drills. Warm up for 10-20 minutes in Zone 1 or at "easy" pace; then spend about 10 minutes on the following drills before finishing the remainder of the run in Zones 1-2 or at "easy" to "conversational" pace.
- Loosening Skips
- Side Skips
- Carioca, or Grapevine with High Knee
- Straight Leg Run
- Butt Kicks

- High Knees
- Ankling
  (see end of chapter for explanation of drills)

Where: Flats (grass, trail or track)

How: Use heart rate, pace or perceived exertion to monitor intensity

Run (Easy with Drill Session 4)

When: Any training phase

Why: To aid recovery, add to your training volume and work on form

What: This is an easy run with a focus on drills. Warm up for 10-20 minutes in Zone 1 or at "easy" pace; then spend about 10 minutes on the following drills before finishing the remainder of the run in Zones 1-2 or at "easy" to "conversational" pace.
- Loosening Skips
- Side Skips
- A Skip
- B Skip
- Straight Leg Run
- Butt Kicks
- High Knees
- Ankling
  (see end of chapter for explanation of drills)

Where: Flats (grass, trail or track)

How: Use heart rate, pace or perceived exertion to monitor intensity

Bike (Pre-race Warmup)

When: Day before a race

Why: To loosen up, check equipment, and scout out the course

What: This is effectively an "active rest day." Your aim is get in a short warm up to check equipment and loosen up.

You will have a lot of energy, especially with the excitement of race week. But remember that today is not the race nor is it a day for an extended workout. Do just enough to get the blood flowing, keeping it in Zone 1 with a few striders.

Stay hydrated and fueled. Eat well, and relax in preparation for the race.

Where: Race course (if possible)

How: Use perceived exertion and pace to monitor intensity

Endurance Workouts

Run (Endurance)

When: All training phases, especially base training

Why: To build the aerobic base by developing the ability to better metabolize fat and spare glycogen (stored carbohydrate) as a long duration energy source

What: Run primarily in Zone 2 or at "conversational" pace for the bulk of the run. Focus on keeping cadence between at least 28-30 left foot strikes per 20 seconds (84-90 per minute).

Where: Flats, hills, treadmill

How: Use heart rate, pace or perceived exertion to monitor intensity

Run (Endurance with Acceleration Striders)

When: All training phases, especially base training

Why: To build the aerobic base and neuromuscular speed

What: Run primarily in Zone 2 or at "conversational" pace. Focus on keeping cadence between at least 28-30 left foot strikes per 20 seconds (84-90 per minute). Throughout the run, throw in 6-8 x short accelerations. Start off easy and gradually pick up your pace until you're at full speed. Hold full speed for up to 10 seconds; then wind it back down. These are "feel good" sprints—you want to feel good going fast. Focus on good form and leg turnover. Run easy for 2-3 minutes between each strider or until you feel fully recovered and ready for the next one. Don't worry about time or heart rate on the striders.

Where: Flats (grass, trail or track)

How: Use heart rate, pace or perceived exertion to monitor intensity

Run (Endurance with Diagonal Striders on Track Infield)

When: All training phases, especially base training

Why: To build the aerobic base and neuromuscular speed

What: Run primarily in Zones 1-2 or at an "easy" to "conversational" pace. Focus on keeping cadence between at least 28-30 left foot strikes per 20 seconds (84-90 per minute). Once you are warmed up, accelerate diagonally across the infield of the track. Start off easy and gradually pick up your pace until you're at full speed. Hold full speed for up to 10 seconds; then wind it back down. These are "feel good" sprints—you want to feel good going fast. Focus on good form and leg turnover. When you reach the corner of the infield, run easy along the width of the field, the length of the field, and the other end of the field. Then start your next diagonal. Run 4-12 x diagonal striders. Don't worry about time or heart rate on the striders.

Where: Track infield

How: Use heart rate, pace or perceived exertion to monitor intensity

Run (Endurance with Short Hills)

When: All training phases, especially base training

Why: To build the aerobic base, neuromuscular speed and power

What: Run primarily in Zones 1-2 or at "easy" to "conversational" pace. Focus on keeping cadence between at least 28-30 left foot strikes per 20 seconds (84-90 per minute). Find a short, steep hill. Once you are warmed up (15-25 minutes), perform 4-12 x 10-second work intervals up the hill at maximum effort. Run at an "easy" pace for about 3-5 minutes in between each hill repeat. When finished with the hills, do the remainder of the run in Zones 1-2 or at "easy" to "conversational" pace. Don't worry about time or heart rate on the hill repeats.

Where: Hills

How: Use heart rate, pace or perceived exertion to monitor intensity

Run (Long)

When: All training phases, especially base training

Why: To build the aerobic base by developing the ability to better metabolize fat and spare glycogen (stored carbohydrate) as a long duration energy source

What: Run primarily in Zone 2 or at "conversational" pace for the bulk of the run. Focus on keeping cadence between at least 28-30 left foot strikes per 20 seconds (84-90 per minute).

Where: Flats, hills, treadmill

How: Use heart rate, pace or perceived exertion to monitor intensity

Run (Long with Fast Finish)

When: All training phases, especially base training

Why: To build the aerobic base and prepare for long course racing effort

What: Run primarily in Zone 2 or at "conversational" pace for the first part of the run. Focus on keeping cadence between at least 28-30 left foot strikes per 20 seconds (84-90 per minute). With about 30-60 minutes left in the run, gradually move into Zones 3-4 or a "comfortably hard" pace. With a mile or two remaining, pick up the pace and push it harder to the finish. Don't worry about heart rate at this point; the goal is to finish fast. By the end, you will have done a three-tier step down of negative splits. This will be a tough workout, but will prepare you for the demands of race day for a longer distance race.

Where: Flats, hills, treadmill

How: Use heart rate, pace or perceived exertion to monitor intensity

Aerobic Tempo Workouts

Run (20-minute Base Tempo)

When: Base training

Why: To build the aerobic base and improve lactate tolerance

What: Once you are thoroughly warmed up (at least 15-20 minutes), up your tempo into Zone 3 or at "comfortably hard" pace for 20 minutes. When finished with the tempo, do the remainder of the run in Zones 1-2 or at "easy" to "conversational" pace. As always, focus on keeping your cadence between at least 28-30 left foot strikes per 20 seconds (84-90 per minute).

Where: Flats, hills, treadmill

How: Use heart rate, pace or perceived exertion to monitor intensity

Run (30-minute Base Tempo)

When: Base training

Why: To build the aerobic base and improve lactate tolerance

What: Once you are thoroughly warmed up (at least 15-20 minutes), up your tempo into Zone 3 or at "comfortably hard" pace for 30 minutes. When finished with the tempo, do the remainder of the run in Zones 1-2 or at "easy" to "conversational" pace. As always, focus on keeping your cadence between at least 28-30 left foot strikes per 20 seconds (84-90 per minute).

Where: Flats, hills, treadmill

How: Use heart rate, pace or perceived exertion to monitor intensity

Run (40-minute Base Tempo)

When: Base training

Why: To build the aerobic base and improve lactate tolerance

What: Once you are thoroughly warmed up (at least 15-20 minutes), up your tempo into Zone 3 or at "comfortably hard" pace for 40 minutes. When finished with the tempo, do the remainder of the run in Zones 1-2 or at "easy" to "conversational" pace. As always, focus on keeping your cadence between at least 28-30 left foot strikes per 20 seconds (84-90 per minute).

Where: Flats, hills, treadmill

How: Use heart rate, pace or perceived exertion to monitor intensity

Threshold Workouts

Run (Sub-LT Cruise Intervals 5/1)

When: Late base training; build training; peak training

Why: To raise the lactate threshold by improving lactate tolerance and decreasing lactate accumulation (which allows you to stay aerobic as faster speeds)

What: Once you are thoroughly warmed up (at least 15-20 minutes), perform up to 12 x 5-min work interval in Zone 4 or at "comfortably hard" pace followed by 1-min recovery interval. When finished with the intervals, do the remainder of run in Zones 1-2 or at "easy" to "conversational" pace ensuring that you complete an adequate warm down (at least 10 minutes). As always, focus on keeping your cadence between at least 28-30 left foot strikes per 20 seconds (84-90 per minute).

Where: Flats, hills, treadmill

How: Use heart rate, pace or perceived exertion to monitor intensity

Run (Sub-LT Cruise Intervals 8/2)

When: Late base training; build training; peak training

Why: To raise the lactate threshold by improving lactate tolerance and decreasing lactate accumulation (which allows you to stay aerobic as faster speeds)

What: Once you are thoroughly warmed up (at least 15-20 minutes), perform up to 7 x 8-min work interval in Zone 4 or at "comfortably hard" pace followed by 2-min recovery interval. When finished with the intervals, do the remainder of run in Zones 1-2 or at "easy" to "conversational" pace ensuring that you complete an adequate warm down (at least 10 minutes). As always, focus on keeping your cadence between at least 28-30 left foot strikes per 20 seconds (84-90 per minute).

Where: Flats, hills, treadmill

How: Use heart rate, pace or perceived exertion to monitor intensity

Run (Sub-LT Cruise Intervals 10/2)

When: Late base training; build training; peak training

Why: To raise the lactate threshold by improving lactate tolerance and decreasing lactate accumulation (which allows you to stay aerobic as faster speeds)

What: Once you are thoroughly warmed up (at least 15-20 minutes), perform up to 6 x 10-min work interval in Zone 4 or at "comfortably hard" pace followed by 2-min recovery interval. When finished with the intervals, do the remainder of run in Zones 1-2 or at "easy" to "conversational" pace ensuring that you complete an adequate warm down (at least 10 minutes). As always, focus on keeping your cadence between at least 28-30 left foot strikes per 20 seconds (84-90 per minute).

Where: Flats, hills, treadmill

How: Use heart rate, pace or perceived exertion to monitor intensity

Run (Sub-LT 20-minute Tempo)

When: Late base training; build training; peak training

Why: To raise the lactate threshold by improving lactate tolerance and decreasing lactate accumulation (which allows you to stay aerobic as faster speeds)

What: Once you are thoroughly warmed up (at least 15-20 minutes), up your tempo into Zone 4 or "comfortably hard" pace for 20 minutes. When finished with the tempo interval, do the remainder of the run in Zones 1-2 or at "easy" to "conversational" pace. As always, focus on keeping your cadence between at least 28-30 left foot strikes per 20 seconds (84-90 per minute).

Where: Flats, hills, treadmill

How: Use heart rate, pace or perceived exertion to monitor intensity

Run (Sub-LT 30-minute Tempo)

When: Late base training; build training; peak training

Why: To raise the lactate threshold by improving lactate tolerance and decreasing lactate accumulation (which allows you to stay aerobic as faster speeds)

What: Once you are thoroughly warmed up (at least 15-20 minutes), up your tempo into Zone 4 or "comfortably hard" pace for 30 minutes. When finished with the tempo interval, do the remainder of the run in Zones 1-2 or at "easy" to "conversational" pace. As always, focus on keeping your cadence between at least 28-30 left foot strikes per 20 seconds (84-90 per minute).

Where: Flats, hills, treadmill

How: Use heart rate, pace or perceived exertion to monitor intensity

Run (Sub-LT 40-minute Tempo)

When: Late base training; build training; peak training

Why: To raise the lactate threshold by improving lactate tolerance and decreasing lactate accumulation (which allows you to stay aerobic as faster speeds)

What: Once you are thoroughly warmed up (at least 15-20 minutes), up your tempo into Zone 4 or "comfortably hard" pace for 40 minutes. When finished with the tempo interval, do the remainder of the run in Zones 1-2 or at "easy" to "conversational" pace. As always, focus on keeping your cadence between at least 28-30 left foot strikes per 20 seconds (84-90 per minute).

Where: Flats, hills, treadmill

How: Use heart rate, pace or perceived exertion to monitor intensity

Run (Sub-LT 60-minute Tempo)

When: Late base training; build training; peak training

Why: To raise the lactate threshold by improving lactate tolerance and decreasing lactate accumulation (which allows you to stay aerobic as faster speeds)

What: Once you are thoroughly warmed up (at least 15-20 minutes), up your tempo into Zone 4 or "comfortably hard" pace for 60 minutes. When finished with the tempo interval, do the remainder of the run in Zones 1-2 or at "easy" to "conversational" pace. As always, focus on keeping your cadence between at least 28-30 left foot strikes per 20 seconds (84-90 per minute).

Where: Flats, hills, treadmill

How: Use heart rate, pace or perceived exertion to monitor intensity

Run (LT Cruise Intervals 5/1)

When: Late base training; build training; peak training

Why: To raise the lactate threshold by improving lactate tolerance and decreasing lactate accumulation (which allows you to stay aerobic as faster speeds)

What: Once you are thoroughly warmed up (at least 15-20 minutes), perform up to 12 x 5-min work interval in Zones 4-5a or at "comfortably hard" pace followed by 1-min recovery interval. When finished with the intervals, do the remainder of run in Zones 1-2 or at "easy" to "conversational" pace ensuring that you complete an adequate warm down (at least 10 minutes). As always, focus on keeping your cadence between at least 28-30 left foot strikes per 20 seconds (84-90 per minute).

Where: Flats, hills, treadmill

How: Use heart rate, pace or perceived exertion to monitor intensity

Run (LT Cruise Intervals 8/2)

When: Late base training; build training; peak training

Why: To raise the lactate threshold by improving lactate tolerance and decreasing lactate accumulation (which allows you to stay aerobic as faster speeds)

What: Once you are thoroughly warmed up (at least 15-20 minutes), perform up to 7 x 8-min work interval in Zones 4-5a or at "comfortably hard" pace followed by 2-min recovery interval. When finished with the intervals, do the remainder of run in Zones 1-2 or at "easy" to "conversational" pace ensuring that you complete an adequate warm down (at least 10 minutes). As always, focus on keeping your cadence between at least 28-30 left foot strikes per 20 seconds (84-90 per minute).

Where: Flats, hills, treadmill

How: Use heart rate, pace or perceived exertion

Run (LT Cruise Intervals 10/2)

When: Late base training; build training; peak training

Why: To raise the lactate threshold by improving lactate tolerance and decreasing lactate accumulation (which allows you to stay aerobic as faster speeds)

What: Once you are thoroughly warmed up (at least 15-20 minutes), perform up to 6 x 10-min work interval in Zones 4-5a or at "comfortably hard" pace followed by 2-min recovery interval. When finished with the intervals, do the remainder of run in Zones 1-2 or at "easy" to "conversational" pace ensuring that you complete an adequate warm down (at least 10 minutes). As always, focus on keeping your cadence between at least 28-30 left foot strikes per 20 seconds (84-90 per minute).

Where: Flats, hills, treadmill

How: Use heart rate, pace or perceived exertion to monitor intensity

Run (LT 20-minute Tempo)

When: Late base training; build training; peak training

Why: To raise the lactate threshold by improving lactate tolerance and decreasing lactate accumulation (which allows you to stay aerobic as faster speeds)

What: Once you are thoroughly warmed up (at least 15-20 minutes), up your tempo into Zones 4-5a or "comfortably hard" pace for 20 minutes. When finished with the tempo interval, do the remainder of the run in Zones 1-2 or at "easy" to "conversational" pace. As always, focus on keeping your cadence between at least 28-30 left foot strikes per 20 seconds (84-90 per minute).

Where: Flats, hills, treadmill

How: Use heart rate, pace or perceived exertion to monitor intensity

Run (LT 30-minute Tempo)

When: Late base training; build training; peak training

Why: To raise the lactate threshold by improving lactate tolerance and decreasing lactate accumulation (which allows you to stay aerobic as faster speeds)

What: Once you are thoroughly warmed up (at least 15-20 minutes), up your tempo into Zones 4-5a or "comfortably hard" pace for 30 minutes. When finished with the tempo interval, do the remainder of the run in Zones 1-2 or at "easy" to "conversational" pace. As always, focus on keeping your cadence between at least 28-30 left foot strikes per 20 seconds (84-90 per minute).

Where: Flats, hills, treadmill

How: Use heart rate, pace or perceived exertion to monitor intensity

Run (LT 40-minute Tempo)

When: Late base training; build training; peak training

Why: To raise the lactate threshold by improving lactate tolerance and decreasing lactate accumulation (which allows you to stay aerobic as faster speeds)

What: Once you are thoroughly warmed up (at least 15-20 minutes), up your tempo into Zones 4-5a or "comfortably hard" pace for 40 minutes. When finished with the tempo interval, do the remainder of the run in Zones 1-2 or at "easy" to "conversational" pace. As always, focus on keeping your cadence between at least 28-30 left foot strikes per 20 seconds (84-90 per minute).

Where: Flats, hills, treadmill

How: Use heart rate, pace or perceived exertion to monitor intensity

Run (LT 60-minute Tempo)

When: Late base training; build training; peak training

Why: To raise the lactate threshold by improving lactate tolerance and decreasing lactate accumulation (which allows you to stay aerobic as faster speeds)

What: Once you are thoroughly warmed up (at least 15-20 minutes), up your tempo into Zones 4-5a or "comfortably hard" pace for 60 minutes. When finished with the tempo interval, do the remainder of the run in Zones 1-2 or at "easy" to "conversational" pace. As always, focus on keeping your cadence between at least 28-30 left foot strikes per 20 seconds (84-90 per minute).

Where: Flats, hills, treadmill

How: Use heart rate, pace or perceived exertion to monitor intensity

Run (LT Track 800s)

When: Late base training; build training; peak training

Why: To raise the lactate threshold by improving lactate tolerance and decreasing lactate accumulation (which allows you to stay aerobic as faster speeds)

What: Once you are thoroughly warmed up (15-25 minutes), perform up to 4-16 x 800-meters in Zones 4-5a or at "comfortably hard" pace with 100-meters easy recovery jog between. If you are using pace, your target time should be right around your functional threshold pace (FTP). When finished with the intervals, do the remainder of the run in Zones 1-2 or at "easy" to "conversational" pace. As always, focus on keeping your cadence between at least 28-30 left foot strikes per 20 seconds (84-90 per minute).

Where: Track, treadmill

How: Use heart rate, pace or perceived exertion to monitor intensity

Run (LT Track 1600s)

When: Late base training; build training; peak training

Why: To raise the lactate threshold by improving lactate tolerance and decreasing lactate accumulation (which allows you to stay aerobic as faster speeds)

What: Once you are thoroughly warmed up (15-25 minutes), perform up to 2-8 x 1600-meters in Zones 4-5a or at "comfortably hard" pace with 200-meters easy recovery jog between. If you are using pace, your target time should be right around your functional threshold pace (FTP). When finished with the intervals, do the remainder of the run in Zones 1-2 or at "easy" to "conversational" pace. As always, focus on keeping your cadence between at least 28-30 left foot strikes per 20 seconds (84-90 per minute).

Where: Track, treadmill

How: Use heart rate, pace or perceived exertion to monitor intensity

Run (LT Mile Repeats)

When: Late base training; build training; peak training

Why: To raise the lactate threshold by improving lactate tolerance and decreasing lactate accumulation (which allows you to stay aerobic as faster speeds)

What: Once you are thoroughly warmed up (15-25 minutes), perform up to 2-8 x 1-mile in Zones 4-5a or at "comfortably hard" pace with 200-meters easy recovery jog between. If you are using pace, your target time should be right around your functional threshold pace (FTP). When finished with the intervals, do the remainder of the run in Zones 1-2 or at "easy" to "conversational" pace. As always, focus on keeping your cadence between at least 28-30 left foot strikes per 20 seconds (84-90 per minute).

Where: Flats, hills, treadmill

How: Use heart rate, pace or perceived exertion

Vo_2 Max Workouts

Run (VO_2 Intervals 3/2)

When: Build training; peak training

Why: To increase the maximal rate of oxygen transport (aerobic capacity or VO2max), build lactate tolerance, and increase anaerobic endurance

What: Once you are thoroughly warmed up (15-25 minutes), perform up to 9 x 3-min work interval in Zone 5b or "uncomfortably hard" pace followed by 2-min recovery interval. When finished with the intervals, do the remainder of the run in Zones 1-2 or at "easy" to "conversational" pace ensuring that you complete an adequate warm down (at least 10 minutes). As always, focus on keeping your cadence between at least 28-30 left foot strikes per 20 seconds (84-90 per minute).

Where: Flats, hills, treadmill

How: Use heart rate, pace or perceived exertion to monitor intensity

Run (VO₂ Intervals 4/3)

When: Build training; peak training

Why: To increase the maximal rate of oxygen transport (aerobic capacity or VO2max), build lactate tolerance, and increase anaerobic endurance

What: Once you are thoroughly warmed up (15-25 minutes), perform up to 7 x 4-min work interval in Zone 5b or "uncomfortably hard" pace followed by 3-min recovery interval. When finished with the intervals, do the remainder of the run in Zones 1-2 or at "easy" to "conversational" pace ensuring that you complete an adequate warm down (at least 10 minutes). As always, focus on keeping your cadence between at least 28-30 left foot strikes per 20 seconds (84-90 per minute).

Where: Flats, hills, treadmill

How: Use heart rate, pace or perceived exertion to monitor intensity

Run (VO₂ Intervals 5/4)

When: Build training; peak training

Why: To increase the maximal rate of oxygen transport (aerobic capacity or VO2max), build lactate tolerance, and increase anaerobic endurance

What: Once you are thoroughly warmed up (15-25 minutes), perform up to 6 x 5-min work interval in Zone 5b or "uncomfortably hard" pace followed by 4-min recovery interval. When finished with the intervals, do the remainder of the run in Zones 1-2 or at "easy" to "conversational" pace ensuring that you complete an adequate warm down (at least 10 minutes). As always, focus on keeping your cadence between at least 28-30 left foot strikes per 20 seconds (84-90 per minute).

Where: Flats, hills, treadmill

How: Use heart rate, pace or perceived exertion to monitor intensity

Run (VO$_2$ Track 800s)

When: Build training; peak training

Why: To increase the maximal rate of oxygen transport (aerobic capacity or VO2max), build lactate tolerance, and increase anaerobic endurance

What: Once you are thoroughly warmed up (15-25 minutes), perform 4-10 x 800-meters in Zone 5b or at "uncomfortably hard" pace with 400-meters easy recovery jog between. When finished with the intervals, do the remainder of the run in Zones 1-2 or at "easy" to "conversational" pace. As always, focus on keeping your cadence between at least 28-30 left foot strikes per 20 seconds (84-90 per minute).

Where: Track, treadmill

How: Use heart rate, pace or perceived exertion to monitor intensity

Anaerobic Capacity Workouts

Run (Speed Reps 1/2)

When: Build training; peak training

Why: To improve the ability to maintain short durations of speed of up to 2 minutes in duration (starts, race surges, finishing kicks)

What: Once you are thoroughly warmed up (15-25 minutes), perform up to 10 x 1-min work interval in Zone 5c or "all out" pace followed by 2-min recovery interval. (Note: heart rate generally takes about 30 seconds to move into target zone so focus on being in Zone 5c over last part of the work interval.) When finished with the intervals, do the remainder of the run at an easy pace (Zones 1-2) ensuring that you complete an adequate warm down (at least 10 minutes). As always, focus on keeping your cadence between at least 28-30 left foot strikes per 20 seconds (84-90 per minute).

Where: Flats, hills, treadmill

How: Use heart rate, pace or perceived exertion to monitor intensity

Run (Speed Reps 2/4)

When: Build training; peak training

Why: To improve the ability to maintain short durations of speed of up to 2 minutes in duration (starts, race surges, kicks)

What: Once you are thoroughly warmed up (15-25 minutes), perform up to 6 x 2-min work interval in Zone 5c or "all out" pace followed by 4-min recovery interval. (Note: heart rate generally takes about 30 seconds to move into target zone so focus on being in Zone 5c over last part of the work interval.) When finished with the intervals, do the remainder of the run at an easy pace (Zones 1-2) ensuring that you complete an adequate warm down (at least 10 minutes). As always, focus on keeping your cadence between at least 28-30 left foot strikes per 20 seconds (84-90 per minute).

Where: Flats, hills, treadmill

How: Use heart rate, pace or perceived exertion to monitor intensity

Run (Track 400s)

When: Build training; peak training

Why: To improve the ability to maintain short durations of speed of up to 2 minutes in duration (starts, race surges, finishing kicks)

What: Once you are thoroughly warmed up (15-25 minutes), run up to 8 x 400-meters in Zone 5c or at "all out" pace followed by 400-meters recovery. When finished with the intervals, do the remainder of the run at an easy pace (Zones 1-2) ensuring that you complete an adequate warm down (at least 10 minutes). As always, focus on keeping your cadence between at least 28-30 left foot strikes per 20 seconds (84-90 per minute).

Where: Track, treadmill

How: Use heart rate, pace or perceived exertion to monitor intensity

Run (Track 400s)

When: Build training; peak training

Why: To improve the ability to maintain short durations of speed of up to 2 minutes in duration (starts, race surges, finishing kicks)

What: Warm up for 20-30 minutes. Run 600 meters in Zone 5c or "all out" pace. When done, do a 100-meter easy recovery jog (on the straightaway). Then immediately go into 12 x 100-meters (on the curve) with an easy jog across the infield to get back to the beginning of the curve in between. The point of this workout is to put you into oxygen debt and keep you there while your body tries to manage the high levels of lactate. You will be spent at the end; be sure to warm down well to clear out the lactate that builds up during this session.

Where: Track

How: Use heart rate, pace or perceived exertion to monitor intensity

Running Drills

Side-to-Side Skip

Running takes place almost exclusively in the sagittal plane (flexion/extension) to propel the runner forward, yet muscles that operate in the frontal plane (abduction/adduction) play an important role as stabilizers. These first two drills build strength and coordination among these stabilizing muscles. For the side-to-side skip, skip side to side by bringing your feet together and then shoulder width apart. Let your arms cross over each other in front of the body as you skip.

Carioca, or Grapevine

Like the side-to-side skips, the carioca or grapevine drill further works the stabilizing muscles that play a secondary but nevertheless vital role in running. As you move sideways, cross one leg over the other in front and then behind. Hold your arms out to the side to begin; as you start to get the hang of the drill, use your arms as you would while running.

Carioca with High Knee

Perform the carioca drill, but now lift your front leg high as you cross over. Continue using the bag leg as usual. Just the front leg goes high.

A Skip

These next drills recruit the primary movers—namely, the glutes and hamstrings—that operate during the active propulsion phase of the run. For the A-skip, skip with high knees. As you bring your leg down, finish with a slight pawing motion as you pull backwards. This pawing motion is often neglected, but is a key element of a powerful stride. Focus on initiating that pull from the glutes as the hamstrings then join in the motion. This will ingrain the backward pulling motion important for running propulsion into your muscle memory. Use the same arm motion during this drill as you use while running.

B Skip

The B-skip is nearly identical to the A skip, but first extends the leg forward. This extension of the leg dynamically stretches the hamstring and then allows you to really emphasize the backward pawing motion as your foot lands on the ground and pulls through. Get into the rhythm of the A and B skips by listening to the pattern of sound your feet make as they contact and scuff the ground, pawing backwards. Use the same arm motion during this drill as you use while running.

Butt Kick

The butt kick drill further conditions and coordinates the glutes and hamstrings for a strong running stride. The butt kick drill should almost feel like a variation of running with high knees (rather than simply kicking backwards). Pull your heels up directly beneath you, keeping the knee, heel and toe up throughout the drill. Use the same arm motion during this drill as you use while running.

High Knee

The high knee drill works the loading phase of the run. The key to performing the drill correctly is to drive the foot down and let it spring back up off the ground (rather than lifting the knees). Use the same arm motion during this drill as you use while running.

Straight Leg Run

The straight leg run reinforces the important pawing motion practiced in the A-skip and B-skip. Start slowly and gradually increase your speed. Avoid the temptation to lean backwards—in other words, keep your upper body perpendicular to the ground as you run with straight legs. As your foot contacts the ground, finish with that same backwards pawing motion as you practiced in the other drills—squeeze the glutes and hamstrings as you pull back on the track.

Ankling

The ankling drill helps facilitate the proper loading and spring during running. Starting at the toe, push the foot down so that the heel barely contacts the ground. The movement can be difficult to learn at first, so begin in slow motion; then gradually pick up the pace and keep the cadence high.

Partner High Knee

Stand so you and your partner face each other. Partner A places their arms into the running position. Partner B holds their hands about an inch in front of Partner A's upper chest (below the shoulders), ready to take the weight of Partner A. Partner A then drops their torso forward—leaning from the ankles—and falls into Partner B's hands.

The lean is slight and the ankles are the pivot point (do not hunch forward at the waist!). Hold this for several seconds to get a feel for this position. Make sure you are not allowing yourself to bend forward at the waist; let your partner hold your weight.

Once you and your partner have traded roles a few times, add the next component of the progression. With Partner A leaning into Partner B, Partner B steps to the side as Partner A carries momentum from the lean into a run for about 10 meters. Be sure to start with a short step to ensure the tall body position with the slight lean is maintained. The key is to carry this body position into the run.

The final component of the progression is the partner high knee drill. Start again with Partner A leaning into Partner B. Now, Partner A drives forward with high knees as Partner B provides resistance while walking/jogging backward. After about 10 meters, Partner B steps to the side, and Partner A carries the form into a run for another 20 meters. The key here is for Partner A to maintain the body position and momentum from the forward lean into the run.

Another variation on the partner high knee drill is to use a running harness. You can either have a partner provide resistance by holding the harness from behind or attach the harness to a tire (no partner required) that you drag behind you.

Achilles Drill

Stand so that you face a wall two feet away. Keep your entire foot on the ground and allow your body to roll forward at the ankle so that you "fall" into the wall. (Use your hands to stop your chest from hitting the wall.)

The goal is to avoid the tendency to push off at the ankle (as you "fall" into the wall). You want to replicate this motion while running. When running, think about keeping the ankle loose.

Single Leg Balance Drill

It's best to perform this drill barefoot.

Firmly ground one foot. Think about spreading the toes and planting the little toe, bit toe and heel as three points of a tripod. This will help you distribute weight equally over your forefoot and rear foot as you establish a solid contact point.

Lift your opposite leg off the ground with a high knee so that the thigh is parallel to the ground.

Now squeeze that glute to bring the elevated leg back so that the calf is parallel with the ground.

Hold this position for 30 seconds. Close your eyes to make it more difficult.

With a partner, you can toss a medicine ball back and forth while in this position. On your own, you can add more instability by standing on a balance disk or rocker board.

Work both legs. Frequency of practice is key to developing improved balance. Do this frequently throughout the day, such as while brushing your teeth or standing in line at the store. This will strengthen the proprioception in your feet and teach your core muscles to work together as you run.

Runner's Toe Touch Drill

It's best to perform this drill barefoot.

Firmly ground one foot. Think about spreading the toes and planting the little toe, bit toe and heel as three points of a tripod. This will help you distribute weight equally over your forefoot and rear foot as you establish a solid contact point.

With one foot planted on the ground, lift your opposite leg off the ground in a high knee position. Stand in a running pose. Now bend at the waist and touch your left foot with your right hand. Return to the standing running pose. Repeat several times. Then do the same on the other side.

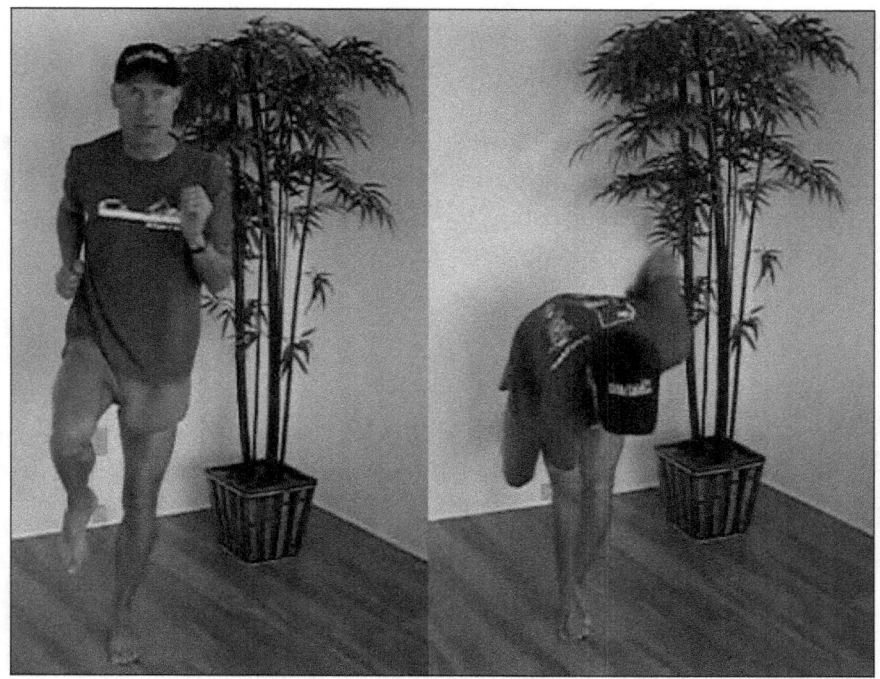

Figure 10-1. Runner's toe touch balance drill

Dynamic Warm Up Activities

High Knee Hurdle Walk

Begin by walking with high knees for 10 to 20 meters. Moving from the high knee walk, now add the hurdle component. Imagine you are stepping over the side of a hurdle as your walk. Drive with your knee and rotate around the hip joint. Do this for 10 to 20 meters.

Straight Leg Walk

For the straight leg walk, keep the leg straight and lift it up as high as you can by contracting the quads and hip flexors. As you bring your foot back to the ground, aim to finish with a slight scuffing or pawing motion. Never go to the point of strain nor force the movement. Only lift the leg as high as you can with comfort.

Backward Walk with Waist Bend

Starting in a standing position, hinge forward at the waist by pushing the butt backward. Return to the standing position, and take a half step backward with one foot. Hinge forward again at the waist. Return to the standing position, and take a half step backward with the other foot. Repeat this motion for about 10 meters to warm up your lower back and hamstrings.

Toe Walk and Heel Walk

For the toe walk, walk 10 to 20 meters on your toes. This will engage the calf muscles.

For the heel walk, walk 10 to 20 on your heels. This will engage the muscles on the front part of your lower leg (i.e. tibialis anterior).

Loosening Skips

Skip lightly while keeping your arms relaxed. Do this for 10 to 20 meters.

Next, add forward arm circles for 10 to 20 meters. Switch to backward arm circles for 10 to 20 meters.

Switch to forward arm circles with both arms for 10 to 20 meters.

Switch to backward arm circles with both arms for 10 to 20 meters.

Finally, open up the chest with a cross-chest arm swing for 10 to 20 meters.

Leg Swings

Leg swings are designed to warm up muscles and increase mobility around the hip joint prior to activity. There are three movement patterns for these leg swings. The first two are based on the spiral-diagonal movement patterns that arise from the way muscles are placed on the skeleton system. These patterns are emphasized in PNF (proprioceptive neuromuscular facilitation) stretching techniques, and mimic normal movement patterns that combine various planes of motion. The third pattern follows the typical flexion/extension pattern through the sagittal plane used while running. As you perform the leg swings, think about actively controlling the movement patterns with particular focus on the glutes.

D1 (diagonal one) Pattern: Stand on your left foot (it is helpful to hold onto something with your left arm, like a wall or fence). Bring your right leg forward and across your body, and point your foot to the right—here, your leg is externally rotated (i.e. your right foot looks like it is kicking a soccer ball). Slowly swing the leg behind and away from your body until your right foot points to the left—as you do this, you are internally rotating the leg. This is the D1 movement pattern for the right leg. Repeat several controlled swings (e.g. 8-12) with the right leg and then do the same on the other side with the left leg.

D2 (diagonal two) Pattern: Stand on your left foot (it is helpful to hold onto something with your left arm, like a wall or fence). Bring your right leg forward and out away from your body with your foot pointing to the left—here, your leg is internally rotated. Slowly swing the leg behind and across your body until your foot is plantar flexed (toes pointed)—as you do this, you are externally rotating the leg. This is the D2 movement pattern for the right leg. Repeat several controlled swings (e.g. 8-12) with the right leg and then switch to do the same with the left leg.

Sagittal Pattern: Stand on your left foot (it is helpful to hold onto something with your left arm, like a wall or fence). With the leg straight, lift it in front of the body. Slowly swing the leg behind the body. This is the forward/backward movement pattern for the right leg. Repeat several controlled swings (e.g. 8-12) with the right leg and then switch to do the same with the left leg.

GLOSSARY

Adenosine triphosphate (ATP)

ATP is a high-energy compound that acts as the basic currency of energy in our bodies. Muscles store ATP in limited amounts which can be quickly tapped for energy. However, the amounts are so limited that any type of activity over a few seconds in duration requires the creation of additional ATP through one of several metabolic pathways (e.g. anaerobic glycolysis or aerobic oxidation).

Aerobic

The term aerobic refers to the type of energy metabolism carried out by your body in the presence of oxygen. Aerobic metabolism, or aerobic oxidation sustains exercise for longer durations of time. The aerobic system uses stored fats, carbohydrates (glycogen), and proteins as energy sources.

As the intensity level of exercise increases, the body must rely more upon anaerobic metabolism to meet its pressing energy needs.

N.B. It is important to recognize that the different types of energy systems used by the body to fuel exercise are not mutually exclusive. They all operate during exercise but to differing degrees depending upon the intensity of the exercise.

Aerobic capacity

Aerobic capacity is a term used synonymously with VO_2max, or maximal oxygen consumption. These terms refer to the highest rate of oxygen transport and use by your body during maximal physical exertion.

VO_2max is expressed through the Fick equation, which multiplies heart rate (HR) by stroke volume (SV) by arteriovenous oxygen difference (a-v O_2 difference): VO_2max (mL/kg/min) = HR (beat/min) x SV (mL/beat) x (a-v O2 difference).

VO_2max can be expressed in absolute terms as liters per minute (L/min), but is typically expressed relative to body weight so that comparisons among individuals can be made. Relative VO_2max is therefore expressed as milliliters per kilogram per minute (mL/kg/min).

Anaerobic

The term anaerobic refers to the type of energy metabolism carried out by your body without oxygen. Anaerobic metabolism, or anaerobic glycolysis is used to meet the body's energy needs at higher levels of intensity. It uses carbohydrates (glycogen or glucose) to rapidly produce energy for the body.

The end product of anaerobic metabolism is lactate, which requires aerobic metabolism (and hence oxygen) to remove from the bloodstream. Any bout of exercise over a few minutes, therefore, cannot be sustained solely through anaerobic metabolism.

N.B. It is important to recognize that the different types of energy systems used by the body to fuel exercise are not mutually exclusive. They all operate during exercise but to differing degrees depending upon the intensity of the exercise.

Arteriovenous oxygen difference (a-v O2 difference)

Oxygenated blood leaves the heart through arteries. As the blood circulates throughout the body, muscles extract some of that oxygen for use in energy production. The a-v O_2 difference reflects the difference between the oxygen concentration in the arteries (leaving the heart) and the remaining oxygen concentration in the veins (returning to the heart).

At rest, the a-v O_2 difference is typically around 5 milliliters of oxygen per deciliter (5 mL O_2/dL), representing a use coefficient of 25 percent. At exercise, the a-v O_2 difference can increase up to around 15 mL O_2/dL with a use coefficient of 75 percent. In other words, more oxygen is extracted by working muscles as the intensity level of oxygen increases.

Base training

Base training refers to the phase, or period of training that primarily works the aerobic system to build endurance and prepare the body for the demands of higher intensity training down the road. Base training is marked by increases in training volume.

Blood pressure

Your blood pressure consists of two numbers: systolic blood pressure (SBP) and diastolic blood pressure (DBP). The systolic blood pressure refers to the pressure exerted on the wall of your arteries when the heart contracts. The diastolic blood pressure refers to the arterial pressure during the relaxation phase of the heart's ventricles.

Typical resting blood pressure is 120/80 (that is, 120 mm Hg for systolic pressure and 80 mm Hg for diastolic pressure). Consistent resting blood pressure readings at or above 140/90 generally constitute high blood pressure, or hypertension.

Build training

The build training phase occurs after base training. Build training is marked by a leveling off or decrease in volume while intensity increases.

Cadence

Cadence refers to the number of revolutions, or cycles per minute. For swimming, cadence refers to the number of swim strokes per minute. For cycling, cadence refers to the number of pedals strokes per minute. For running, cadence refers to the number of foot strikes per minute.

Cardiac output (Q)

Cardiac output refers to the volume of blood pumped by the heart each minute. Cardiac output (abbreviated Q with a dot over it, or Q-dot) is calculated by multiplying heart rate (HR) by stroke volume (SV): Q = HR x SV.

Central adaptations

This term refers to the general adaptations that occur to the central respiratory and cardiovascular systems as the result of training.

Duration

Training duration refers to the amount of time of a training session. The frequency of training sessions plus the duration of those training sessions comprise training volume.

Fast-twitch

Fast-twitch muscle fibers—also called Type IIx—contract more quickly and with more force than any other fiber type. They contribute substantially to shorter bursts of speed and do so through anaerobic energy production pathways. When a chicken is startled and flaps its wings to get away from a perceived threat, it recruits those fast-twitch fibers in the chest to move quickly. In contrast, the slow-twitch muscle fibers in the chicken's legs are recruited for the long duration task of walking around the farmyard all day long.

FITT

This is an acronym that stands for frequency (how often), intensity (how hard), time (how long), and type (of activity). It is used to ensure you take into account these four parameters in designing a workout plan.

Flexibility

Flexibility refers to the range of motion around joints.

Frequency

Training frequency refers to the number of training sessions done per week. The frequency of training sessions plus the duration of those training sessions comprise training volume.

Functional strength

Functional strength refers to strength that directly benefits sport specific movements and activities.

Functional threshold pace (FTPa)

The functional threshold pace (FTPa) is your pace at lactate threshold.

General adaptation syndrome (GAS)

When you train, you introduce a stimulus, or "stress" to your body. This is followed by a "response" from the body which leads to a physiological "adaptation." Hungarian biologist Hans Selye called this stress-response-adaptation process the general adaptation syndrome (GAS).

Goals

Goals refer to desired results towards which achievement is directed. Goals can be categorized as performance goals, process goals, or outcome goals. While outcome goals provide long-term motivation and many long-term goals take this form, performance and process goals help athletes focus on what needs to be done in the intermediate and short-term, such as in the moment of the race.

Performance goals: Performance goals have to do with achieving a certain time (e.g., breaking 10 hours in the Ironman, running a 40-minute 10K).

Process goals: Process goals have to do with how you compete (e.g., keep my cadence high during the last half of my Ironman run).

Outcome goals: Outcome goals have to do with placement in a race (e.g., finishing on the podium).

Heart rate (HR)

Heart rate refers to the number of times your heart beats per minute.

Heart rate training zones

Heart rate training zones are ranges used for exercise prescription. They can be percentages based on, among other things, VO2max, VO2 Reserve, HRmax, HR Reserve, LTHR, among others. The heart rate training zones generally used by Alp Fitness include seven levels that correspond to percentages of lactate threshold heart rate (LTHR).

Intensity

Training intensity refers to the effort put forth during a training session, as measured through effort, exertion, speed, power, etc. Training intensity is one of two key axes around which your training revolves—the other is volume.

Intermediate fast-twitch

Intermediate fast-twich, or Type IIa muscle fibers. These muscle fibers possess some of the aerobic characteristics of the slow-twitch fibers as well as some of the increased contractile capability of the fast-twitch fibers.

Interval training

In general terms, interval training refers to the use of higher intensity work bouts, or work intervals interspersed with recovery intervals or rest intervals. The length of the work and recovery intervals can vary depending upon what training effect you are trying to achieve.

Note that running coach Jack Daniels uses the term "intervals" in a more specific way to refer only to VO_2max or race pace intervals of 3 to 5 minutes in duration. He uses the term reps (repetitions) to refer to work periods of less than 2 minutes in duration at highest intensity.

Lactate threshold (LT)

Lactate is a by-product of your body's energy production and the lactate threshold (LT) can be thought of as the boundary line between aerobic work and anaerobic work. Workloads above the lactate threshold can only be sustained for up to a few minutes before the body must slow down. Workloads right at the lactate threshold can generally be maintained for about an hour or even two. Workloads below the lactate threshold can be maintained much longer.

In physiological terms, the lactate threshold (LT) refers to the intensity at which the rate of appearance of lactate in the blood exceeds the rate of its disappearance. In other words, when you reach lactate threshold, your bloodstream begins to accumulate more lactate than it can clear. The presence of lactate in your blood isn't a problem in and of itself. However, accompanying the lactate are positively charged hydrogen atoms that make the blood acidic. This acidic environment contributes to muscle fatigue and that burning sensation you feel when you're exercising at a high intensity.

An important effect of endurance training is to 'raise your lactate threshold.' Whereas before training you could run, say, 7 minutes per mile while at LT, after training the same pace would represent an intensity level below your LT. This means that you would be able to go faster at a lower level of effort.

Lactate threshold heart rate (LTHR)

Your lactate threshold heart rate (LTHR) is the heart rate that corresponds to your lactate threshold (LT). It is specific to the activity, so you will have a different LTHR for running, cycling, swimming, etc. An athlete's LTHR for cycling is typically 5 to 10 beats lower than that athlete's LTHR for running, so it is possible to estimate one from the other if sport specific tests are not available for both.

Macrocycle

Macrocycle refers to the period of time on which a season's training plan is based. A macrocycle typically corresponds to a calendar year or the length of time dedicated to a particular training plan (e.g. 24 weeks). The macrocycle is divided into smaller phases of about one to six weeks in length called mesocycles.

Mesocycle

Mesocycle refers to a training period comprised of several microcycles. Each mesocycle has a particular training focus, and typically lasts from two to six weeks.

Microcycle

Microcycle refers to a training "week." This typically corresponds to a seven day calendar week. It is quite possible to use microcycles of, say, 10 days instead of the seven day week. Such an approach could have advantages for some athletes, but for many it is easier to schedule a microcycle around the typical calendar week.

Muscle fibers

Muscle fibers are muscle cells. They come in three types: Type I (slow-twitch), Type IIx (fast-twitch), and Type IIa (intermediate fast-twitch).

Overload principle

The overload principle states that any new training gain requires a greater amount of training stress. It is important to apply the appropriate amount of stress to overload the system without overreaching or overtraining. For sport specific improvements, the overload principle must also be coupled with the principle of specificity.

Overreaching

Overreaching involves the accumulation of an amount of stress that causes a temporary decrease in performance without showing the signs of overtraining. If overreaching continues long enough without adequate recovery, overtraining can result.

Overtraining

Overtraining refers to the accumulation of too much stress (training or other types of stress) that leads to extreme fatigue (physical and mental). Overtraining occurs when overreaching is carried too far without adequate recovery. With overtraining, the athlete has dug him/herself a hole that may take several weeks to get out of. Extreme cases can be season ending. Overtraining is obviously to be avoided and the administration of an appropriate training plan can help the athlete use the overload principle for performance gains without overtraining.

Peak training

The peak training phase occurs prior to the athlete's key race or races of the season. It occurs after base training has laid a strong aerobic foundation, and it involves a reduction in training volume along with an increase in training intensity to allow the athlete to achieve a high level of fitness for optimal performance.

Peripheral adaptation

This term refers to the physiological adaptations that occur in specific muscle groups as the result of training.

Periodization

Periodization refers to the structuring of training into phases, or periods—such as a base training phase, build phase, race phase, peak training period and so forth. The first use of periodization in training is associated with Tudor Bompa.

Rating of perceived exertion (RPE)

A rating of perceived exertion is a subjective assessment of the intensity level at which one is working. The most common RPE scales are Borg RPE scale (6-20) or Borg category-ratio scale (0-10).

Recovery interval

A recovery interval refers to the time between work bouts in interval training. With a recovery interval (rather than a rest interval), you continue to move but at a slower pace to allow some recovery before the next work interval.

Rest interval

A rest interval refers to the time between work bouts in interval training. A rest interval (rather than a recovery interval) entails a break from activity.

Reversibility

The principle of reversibility states that inactivity leads to performance decline. Performance gains are reversed when the athlete ceases to train at a given level.

Send-off time

In swimming, a send-off time is used during interval training. It includes both the swimmer's swim time plus rest time. For example, let's say you have a set of 10 x 100 where you aim to swim each 100 in about 1:30 with a rest interval of about 15 seconds. In this case, your send-off time would be 1:45, which means you leave the wall every 1:45 for your next 100.

Slow-twitch

Slow-twitch muscle fibers—also called Type I—contract more slowly, just as the name implies. They are built to bring in oxygen and maximize the production of energy through the aerobic pathway. To those ends, they contain a greater number of capillaries and proteins called myoglobin to carry oxygen into the cells, along with a greater number of mitochondria which act as cellular factories for aerobic energy production. The iron-rich pigments associated with myoglobin are responsible for the color of dark meat.

Specificity

The principle of specificity states that training adaptations are specific to the system worked. For example, to improve running performance, one must run rather than swim. It also means that within a given sport, the type of training needs to be geared for the type of racing to be done or performance gains desired.

Stroke volume (SV)

Stroke volume refers to the amount of blood your heart—specifically, your left ventricle—ejects when it contracts.

Tapering

Tapering refers to a decrease in training volume prior to a key race to rest and sharpen the athlete for competition.

Threshold pace

Threshold pace (T-pace) is your pace at lactate threshold.

Training load

The training load is the sum total of training stress thrown at your body in its various forms during training, including both training volume plus training intensity.

Training plan

A training plan provides an organized schedule to help you reach your fitness/competition goals. It uses periodization to maximize training effects according to the overload principle, specificity principle, and other factors that impact progression toward improved performance.

Training zones

Training zones refer to intensity levels used during exercise. Training zones can be based on heart rate, power, velocity, ratings of perceived exertion or some other measurement of work capacity.

Ventilatory threshold (VT)

Ventilatory threshold refers to the point at which breathing first becomes labored during exercise of increasing intensity. It corresponds closely with lactate threshold (LT).

VO_2max

VO_2max (also known as maximal oxygen consumption, or aerobic capacity) refers to the highest rate of oxygen transport and use by your body during maximal physical exertion.

VO_2max is expressed through the Fick equation, which multiplies heart rate (HR) by stroke volume (SV) by arteriovenous oxygen difference (a-v O_2 difference): VO_2max (mL/kg/min) = HR (beat/min) x SV (mL/beat) x (a-v O_2 difference).

VO_2max can be expressed in absolute terms as liters per minute (L/min), but is typically expressed relative to body weight so that comparisons among individuals can be made. Relative VO_2max is therefore expressed as milliliters per kilogram per minute (mL/kg/min).

Volume

Training volume refers to the amount of training done per week. The frequency of training sessions plus the duration of those training sessions comprise training volume. Training volume is one of two key axes around which your training revolves—the other is intensity.

Warmdown

The warmdown, or cooldown period involves a transition from the exercise session back to a resting level. It involves low-level activity to clear lactate from the blood while allowing the heart rate, blood pressure, and respiration rate to lower.

Work interval

A work interval, or work bout refers to the time spent in the target training zone in interval training. Work intervals are interspersed with recovery intervals.

Warmup

The warm up period involves a gradual transition from rest to higher intensity exercise. It involves gradually warming up the body temperature through low-level activity.

About the Author

Adam Hodges, PhD, is a multisport athlete and coach with credentials from USA Triathlon and the American College of Sports Medicine. In addition to coaching multisport athletes, he has coached high school cross country and track runners in California and masters swimmers in Colorado. As a USAT All-American triathlete, he has competed in the ITU World Triathlon Championships, the ITU World Duathlon Championships, and the Ironman World Championships in Hawaii. As a masters runner, he has won a series title in the XTERRA SoCal Trail Series. He began running and competing in triathlons in his youth and enjoys passing on the knowledge and experience he has gained over the years to both new and experienced athletes seeking to maximize enjoyment, competitiveness, and longevity in the sport.

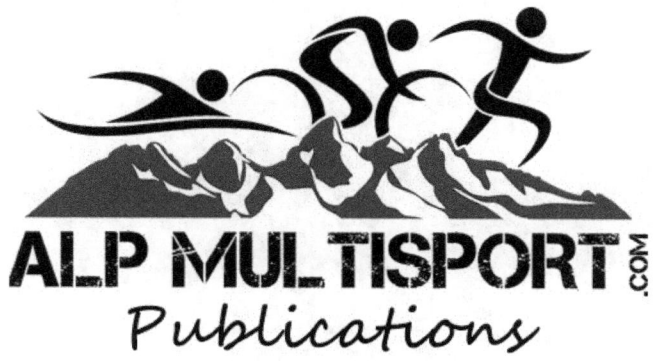

Visit the Alp Fitness website for videos, articles, and training resources to help you train smart!

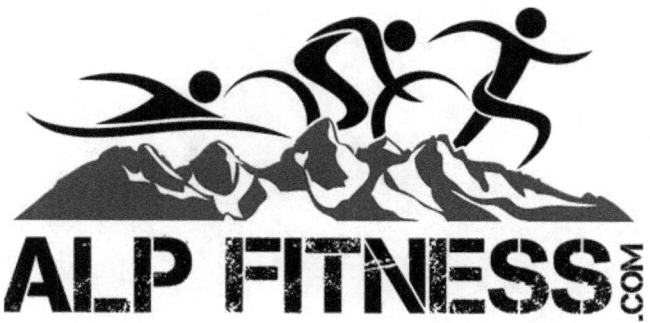

www.ingramcontent.com/pod-product-compliance
Lightning Source LLC
LaVergne TN
LVHW051546070426
835507LV00021B/2440